Beyond PPE:

A Naturopathic Approach To COVID-19

Dr. Vanessa Edwards ND, LAc., MT

Beyond PPE: A Naturopathic Approach To COVID-19

Beyond PPE:
A Naturopathic Approach To COVID-19
©2020 by Dr. Vanessa Edwards
All rights reserved
Printed in the United States of America

Editor: Mrs. Patricia Roberts
Editor: (fiverr-article_h0tpen)
Graphic Design: Ms. Janell Wray

Dr. Vanessa Edwards
Water of Life Naturopathic Healthcare
4421 Salem Ave Dayton OH 45416
www.vedwardsnd.com
ISBN: 978-1-7335615-1-8

Unless otherwise noted, all scripture quotations are taken from the King James Version or New American Standard Version of the Bible.

The material contained in this book is provided for informational purposes only. It is not intended to diagnose, provide medical advice, or take the place of medical advice and treatment from your physician. Readers are advised to consult with a qualified healthcare professional regarding treatment of their specific medical problems. The author is not responsible for any possible consequences from any person reading or following the information in this book. If taking prescription medications, they should consult their physicians and not take themselves off medicines without a physician's proper supervision.

Dedicated To

**Those Who Have Lost
Loved Ones Due To The
2019-2020 COVID-19
Pandemic**

CONTENTS

Introduction

Part 1
Chapter

Part 2
How Creation Prepared Us for COVID-19

Chapter

Part 3

Chapter

Introduction

In the beginning, God...what a statement. When there was nothing, there was God.

The Coronavirus, SARS CoV2, the source of the 2019 pandemic, has been plaguing the world since the end of 2019. Twenty-three million people have been infected with the virus and over eight hundred thousand have lost their lives. Many researchers and scientists are trying to come up with a vaccine or searching for a cure. The question we must ask is, is the virus the invisible enemy?

When I first started hearing about the Coronavirus, I immediately compared the statistics of the virus to influenza. I didn't think it was such a big deal. Then upon further investigation, I began to see the cause of the urgency. This led me to look for evidence-based research that would optimize the Immune system. As I was going through multiple research studies and papers, a friend invited me over to her home to catch up, since we hadn't seen each other in a while due to the stay at home order. We were sitting outside on her deck social distancing, of course sharing and catching up. As we were discussing, the topic of the pandemic came up. She made a statement that I just couldn't get out of my mind, "the problem with this virus is we just don't know who will get it and be asymptomatic and who will get it and have serious side effects." I was in the process of writing this book when this statement was made. As I continued to look at the research, some things began to be really clear. There was a correlation between nutrient deficiencies and how the body responds to viruses. This led me to ask a different question, can nutrient deficiencies play a part in how a person's immune system responds to viruses? Could nutrient sufficiency be the reason why some people are able to mount a correct response to the virus with either having no symptoms or mild symptoms that can be managed at home, compared to those who have an exaggerated or hyper-immune response and have to be hospitalized?

I have spent countless hours combing through research papers and articles and have found evidence-based natural approaches that can help optimize the immune system, and I would like to share these findings with you. Take a journey with me as we look at the creation account in Genesis and see how God gives us ways to support

our immune system during a
pandemic.

CHAPTER 1

How COVID-19 began

History

Coronaviruses are not new; these viruses make up a large group of single-stranded RNA viruses. They are common among mammals and birds. There are actually seven known coronaviruses that affect the human species. Coronaviruses have been known to cause respiratory and gastrointestinal symptoms. The respiratory symptoms caused by Coronaviruses can range from common cold-like symptoms to mild flu-like symptoms, to severe pneumonia that needs ventilatory support. In December 2019, in

1

Wuhan, China, a new strain of the Coronavirus causing pneumonia and death was identified. It was named SARS-CoV2 by the Coronaviridae Study Group of the International Committee on Taxonomy of Viruses because it causes severe acute respiratory syndrome (ARDS) and is 79% genetically similar to SARS-CoV. SARS-CoV caused an outbreak of severe acute respiratory distress in 2002-2003. It is also similar to MERS-CoV, which is the middle Eastern Coronavirus, which also led to pneumonia. It was later named COVID-19. COVID-19 is new to the human immune system; therefore, you may also hear the name "novel" Coronavirus. Because this virus is new to the human immune system, we do not have pre-existing natural immunity against it. It has been hypothesized that this is the reason it has the ability to spread so rapidly. Despite the genetic similarities of COVID-19 to SARS-CoV and MERS-CoV, there are differences in the clinical characteristics. These differences include being 1,000 times more infectious than SARS-CoV; COVID-19 affects the gastrointestinal area at a lower rate; more patients have mild symptoms or express no symptoms at all and are carriers of the virus. The high rate of carriers with no symptoms (asymptomatic) makes the Coronavirus more difficult to contain.

Origin of Coronavirus

In May, retrospective reviews of medical records and CT scans are showing that the Coronavirus may have been circulating in Rome prior to the outbreak in China. Data were collected from patients that were admitted into the ICU for flu-like complications between November 1, 2019 to February 19, 2020.

Results showed that two patients CT imaging features were consistent with COVID-19, and they tested negative for influenza A and B viruses. One patient was admitted at the end of November and the other patient was admitted in the early part of January. Neither patient survived. In France, the first reported case was diagnosed in January but a test done on stored respiratory samples of a patient hospitalized in December was positive for COVID-19. This information has caused concerns about the initial location of the spread of Coronavirus coming out of China.

CHAPTER 2

What Is A Pandemic?

The word pandemic comes from two Greek words *pan* and *demos*, which means "all people." According to the World Health Organization (WHO), a pandemic is the worldwide spread of a new disease. On March 11, 2020, the (WHO) declared COVID-19 a pandemic.

Many times, the words pandemic, epidemic, endemic and outbreak are used interchangeably, but they all have different meanings:

• **Epidemic**- A rapid spread of disease that affects a large number of people within a community,

5

population, or region over a short
period of time.

• **Pandemic**- An epidemic of an
infectious disease that spreads over
multiple countries or continents,
affecting a substantial number of
people.

• **Endemic**- A disease regularly
found among a particular people or
country.

• **Outbreak**- A sudden increase
or rise in the number of
occurrences of a disease in a
particular time and place. It may
affect a small and localized group or
impact thousands of people across
an entire continent

CHAPTER 3

How Taiwan responded to the Pandemic

Taiwan was predicted to have the second-highest number of Covid-19 cases. Due to close proximity to China, and because of the 23 million citizens of Taiwan, 850,000 of them live in China, and 404,000 work in China. Yet, as of July 19, 2020, there have only been 455 confirmed cases and only 7 deaths. Out of 14.3 million cases worldwide, how has Taiwan kept their exposure and death rates so low? When I was made aware of these numbers, I went in search of answers.

It seems as though Taiwan learned several strategies that helped with

7

the containment of infectious diseases from previous experience with the SARS 2003 pandemic and H1N1 flu pandemic in 2009. Those lessons helped Taiwan take control of the spread of COVID-19 before it could take thousands of their residence lives. President Tsai Ing-Wen, of Taiwan stated in her article for Time Magazine on April 16, 2020, "Taiwan's success is no coincidence. The most fundamental element of the Taiwan model is transparency: transparency between the authorities and the public in Taiwan and transparency between Taiwan and the international community. The Taiwan model, which is one of the most effective in the world, is the product of a democratic system."

Leadership

The Vice-President of Taiwan, Dr. Chen Chien-Jen, is a graduate of Johns Hopkins Bloomberg School of Public Health, located in Maryland. Vice President Chen graduated with a Doctor of Science degree in epidemiology and human genetics. The insights he gained during the SARS pandemic played an epic role in Taiwan's response to COVID-19. Some may say he was appointed (chosen) for *such a time as this.*

Timely response / Strategies implemented

Taiwan's epidemic prevention system consisted of rapid response, early deployment, swift decision making, thorough implementation, coordinated resource distribution, transparent information and advanced technology.

One strategy they learned was the importance of continuous monitoring of emerging infectious diseases worldwide. On December 31, 2019, Taiwan's CDC learned from online sources that Wuhan, China, had seven atypical pneumonia cases. They realized that these atypical pneumonia cases were serious, sudden, unusual and incidental events that required immediate attention.

Timeline Response below:

January 2- Taiwan informed the World Health Organization and China's CDC concerning pneumonia cases. Their hospitals infection control department was strengthened.

January 5- Organized advisory committee regarding this atypical pneumonia

January 7- Chinese national ships and cruise ships prohibited from entering Taiwan

January 15- COVID-19 classified as an infectious disease by Taiwan's CDC

January 20- The president of Taiwan held an emergency meeting on COVID-19, addressing containment, outbreak, relief and economic stimulus

January 21- First confirmed case reported. Level 3 travel notice for Wuhan implemented

March 21- Level 3 travel notice implemented for all countries

April 1- Social distancing; encouragemed to wear masks in crowds; the number of people able to gather at temples, national parks, hotels, night markets and shopping centers were reduced

April 16- The average daily production of surgical face masks had increased from 1.9 million to 16 million. Masks allocated to every citizen.

Other strategies implemented by Taiwan:

Border Quarantine

- Non-Residence travelers entering Taiwan: Prior to reserving flights, passengers had to have a health screening and hotel reservations for a 14-day quarantine. Designated Taxis or rental cars were used to transport them to the hotel
- Residence entering Taiwan were quarantined at home or a place away from family and friends for 14 days.

Each passenger entering Taiwan had to undergo health screenings and temperature checks. Those quarantined were visited 1-2 times a day by health officers to make sure they were compliant. They also used electronic security monitors to provide health care and support to those in isolation. This electronic system was also used to alert those leaving the range of quarantine or isolation. If a person had COVID-19 symptoms, they were transported to the hospital by ambulance.

Home quarantine

If a person was ordered to home quarantine by the government, they were provided with a 24hr 7 days a week hotline for health care. They received meal delivery, garbage collection services, and financial assistance for 14 days.

Social distancing

Social distancing was required—1.5 meters indoors or 1-meter outdoors—which is equivalent to 5 feet and 4.5 feet, respectively. Residence went to work and school while practicing social distancing. They are encouraged to only go out for essential needs and large gatherings are discouraged.

Testing

Testing was focused on those who were suspected of having COVID-19 and anyone who came in contact with them. They felt this was a more efficient and cost-effective way to test. Over 60,000 people suspected of having the virus and their contacts have been tested and of that 60,000 only 428 people tested positive as of April 24th.

Contact Tracing

CDC officers were used to help in tracing anyone a person who had tested positive came in contact with in the previous 14 days. Because it may be difficult for a person to recall every place he or she went 14 days prior to them getting ill, Taiwan enlisted the use of telecommunication records. Mobile phone records were used to confirm the footprints of a persons previous 14 days. They also used the National Health Insurance Administration and the Immigration Department to verify hospitals, clinic visits and international travel.

Personal Protective Equipment

Adequate supplies of PPE were available to healthcare workers and non-healthcare workers. Masks were allocated to every citizen.

Taiwan's case numbers were far fewer than the initial model's prediction, in part because the government responded quickly and instituted specific approaches for case identification, containment, and resource allocation to protect the public health.

CHAPTER 4

United States Response To COVID-19

February 9, 2018- President Trump signs bill to cut $1.35 billion in funding for Prevention and Public Health

January 1, 2020- World Health Organization requested information concerning atypical pneumonia cases in Wuhan China

January 3- China provided WHO with information regarding atypical pneumonia cases in Wuhan China

January 20- CDC announced US airports would screen for Coronavirus

January 21- First confirmed case in the United States; travelers from Hubei Province of China. Human to Human spread of Coronavirus confirmed.

January 29- President Trump announced the formation of the President's Coronavirus Task Force

January 31- Secretary of Health and Human Services declared the Coronavirus as a public health emergency. Entry of foreign nationals who had been in certain jurisdictions the prior 14 days where COVID-19 outbreaks occurred was suspended. These areas were China, Iran, and Schengen (26 European countries) (whitehouse.gov)

February 2- US places restrictions on non-US travelers from China entering the US

February (the month of Feb.)- 139,305 travelers arrived to the US from Italy and 1.74 million from Schengen countries (26 European countries), where the outbreak was spreading rapidly, according to the CDC.

February 6- first confirmed US death from the virus

Late February-Mid March (3-week period)- the number of US cases increased 1,000-fold

March 6-21- passengers on cruise ship tested positive for Coronavirus

March 11- World Health Organization (WHO) declared COVID-19 as a pandemic

March 13- President Trump declared COVID-19 a national emergency

March 14- CDC director issued a no sail order for cruise ships, suspending operations in US waters, BUT this order did not go into effect until **April 15**

March 16- Social distancing guidelines given

March 18- CDC reports all ages at risk

March 21- Treasury department and Internal Revenue Service extended filing dates from April 15 to July 15

March 27- President Trump signs 2 trillion-dollar stimulus package

April 3- CDC issued guidance on cloth faced coverings in public areas to reduce the spread

April 6- World health organization (WHO) put out a statement that said, "there is no evidence that wearing a mask (whether medical or other types) by healthy persons in the wider community setting, including universal community masking, can prevent them from infection with respiratory viruses, including COVID-19."

April 6- President Trump agreed to allow the US Navy's 1,000-bed hospital ship, Comfort, to be used to treat patients with Coronavirus in New York

April 9- Student loans deferred for 90 days

April 14- All 50 states have reported cases of Coronavirus

April 20- States announce plans to reopen

April 23- $320 billion allotted for small businesses

April 28- 1 million confirmed cases in the US

May 25- Memorial Day weekend gatherings

May 27- Death toll more than 100,000

May 29- US ends relationship with WHO

May 31- Concerns raised with protest over George Floyd's death— no social distancing

June 11- 2 million confirmed cases in US

June 22- Study by Science Translation Medicine suggested that 80% of Americans who sought care for flu-like illnesses in March went undetected for COVID-19

July 2- President Trump says, "I'm all for mask." He maintained that there was no need to make mask wearing mandatory. John Hopkins reported 2.7 million confirmed cases and 128,000 deaths

July 10- More than 20 states require wearing a mask in public

July 17- President Trump disagrees with CDC's suggestion of making masks mandatory for 4-8 weeks to get Coronavirus under control.

September 8- 34 candidate vaccines under clinical evaluation; 145 vaccines under preclinical evaluation

End of September- The number of new COVID-19 cases/day begin to increase

October 2- President Trump and First Lady test positive for COVID-19

November 3- 9.42 million cases and 232,000 deaths

CHAPTER 5

How the virus is transmitted

The route of transmission of the SARS-CoV2 virus is by human to human contact. Live virus has been found in the nose, mouth, and respiratory droplets—it is transmitted through aerosol droplets. Therefore, when a person coughs, sneezes, or talks and respiratory droplets are released, it can be inhaled by another person, leading to transmission if the droplets contain the virus. Touching contaminated objects and then touching your mouth, nose, or eyes is also a common way the virus is transmitted. The virus has been shown to remain viable on stainless steel and plastic for up to 3 days.

Ten years ago, an observational study was done involving 26 medical students. All students had completed a 4-hour infection control course sometime within the year. They had been educated on the importance of hand hygiene, aseptic techniques, standard precautions, and transmission-based precautions. They were videotaped during a 2-hour lecture. During this lecture, the students touched their faces 2,346 times, which is approximately 23 times an hour.

Mucosal areas of the face touched

- Mouth-31%
- Nose- 27%
- Eyes- 6%

As a precaution, if you touch your
mask, wash or sanitize your hands.

CHAPTER 6

Signs and Symptoms

Symptoms may appear 2-14 days afterexposure

- Dry cough
- Fatigue
- Fever
- Shortness of breath
- Loss of appetite
- Nasal congestion
- Body aches
- Sore throat
- COVID toes
- Diarrhea
- Nausea
- Loss of smell

- Loss of taste
- Headache
- Chills
- Rash
- Asymptomatic(no symptoms)

Complications

- Acute respiratory failure (ARF)
- Acute respiratory distress syndrome (ARDS)
- Acute liver injury
- Acute cardiac injury
- Acute kidney injury
- Pneumonia
- Septic shock
- Miscarriages
- Blood clots
- Disseminated intravascular coagulation

- Rhabdomyolysis (rapid breakdown of skeletal muscle)

Pneumonia and acute respiratory illnesses have been seen among many of the patients hospitalized due to COVID-19. CT scans show lesions on both lungs, which often leads to death.

Who is at risk for having serious complications from COVID-19

Advanced age
Darker-skinned population
Males
Pregnant women
Smokers

Those with:
Hypertension
Diabetes
Obesity

CHAPTER 7

How The Body Fights Coronavirus

The Coronavirus is a double-stranded RNA virus that has spike proteins that look like crowns. This is where it got its name; corona means crown.

When a person comes in contact with the Coronavirus, it enters the body and attaches to receptors located in the lungs, gastrointestinal tract, kidney, heart, bladder, pancreas, nose, and placenta. The receptors that the virus attaches to are called angiotensin converting enzymes 2 (ACE2). The Coronavirus uses its spike proteins to attach to the ACE2 receptors. Once the virus attaches to the receptors, it enters the cell and begins to replicate or reproduce more viruses. The stress of viral replication leads to cell damage and cell death, which in turn, triggers the body to send signals that alert the immune system—the defense system—to initiate an antiviral response. There are several factors involved in the antiviral response. White blood cells are activated to identify and kill the virus. Proinflammatory cytokines and chemokines are released to suppress viral replication and prevent the disease from becoming severe. The SARS CoV2 virus has several mechanisms that prevent the body from stopping it from replicating. If the body is unable to stop the virus from replicating, more and more cytokine and chemokines are released. This causes the body to undergo oxidative stress: oxidative stress is when reactive oxygen species (ROS) are high and antioxidant (against oxidation) levels are low. Antioxidants protect the body from (ROS), which cause tissue damage. When reactive oxygen species levels are high and antioxidants levels are low, this leads to a hyperinflammatory response or a cytokine storm. The cytokine storm causes widespread inflammation and can lead to COVID-19 ARDS (acute respiratory distress). When a person begins to experience ARDS, this can be a potentially life-threatening event and at this point, most patients are put on a ventilator.

CHAPTER 8

Children's immune response to the Coronavirus

Data was collected on 68 children that tested positive for COVID-19 from March to May 2020 in Morocco. The age range of the kids was 1 month to 15 years old. Five of the kids had pre-existing conditions; three had asthma, one was diabetic, and one had heart disease and Down syndrome. Forty-five of the kids were asymptomatic, including the five that had preexisting conditions. The other kids had one or more of the following symptoms: nasal congestion/rhinorrhea, fever, dry cough, diarrhea/vomiting, loss of smell or taste. None of the 68 children became severely or critically ill. Several labs were done on the children, the main abnormalities found were seen in the CBC panel. Four of the patients were anemic, 94% of the children had normal white blood cell (WBC) counts—cells that help your body defend itself. Three had low levels of WBC and 1 had elevated levels. The inflammatory markers and coagulation markers were normal in the majority of the cases.

When comparing the lab work of adults who were positive for covid-19 to children, the opposite is seen with the WBC count in adults. Elevated leukocytes and neutrophil counts were common in patients with unfavorable progression of COVID-19. An elevated neutrophil count is indicative of a bacterial infection on top of the viral infection.

Low lymphocyte counts were only seen in 2 of the children that were positive for the Coronavirus. In comparison, a study showed that 80% of the adults that were positive for COVID-19 and critically ill had low lymphocyte counts. Another author reported that only 25% of the patients with mild COVID-19 cases had low lymphocyte levels. These findings of lymphopenia may correlate with the severity of the COVID-19 infection. This may be due to the fact that vitamin C is stored in lymphocytes. Vitamin C increases glutathione in lymphocytes. Glutathione is one of the major antioxidants in the body; its benefits will be discussed in chapter 11.

Similar findings were seen in China. Out of 44,672 confirmed cases, only 2.1% of the positive cases were less than 19 years old. Comparable similarities were reported during the SARS and MERS outbreaks. Children were affected less than adults and had milder symptoms and better outcomes than adults.

Part 2

Genesis 1:1-5

*In the beginning, God created
the heavens and the earth. The
earth was formless and void,
and darkness was over the
surface of the deep, and the
Spirit of God was moving over
the surface of the waters.
Then God said, "Let there be
light," and there was light. God
saw that the light was good, and
God separated the light from the
darkness.
God called the light day and the
darkness He called night. And
there was evening and there
was morning one day.*

CHAPTER 9
DAY 1

Melatonin Beyond A Good Night's Sleep

Genesis 1:1 says, "In the beginning, God created the heavens and the earth." Let's take a look at the creation account and see how it's relevant to dealing with a pandemic. But before we do that, let's look at the definition of created. In Hebrew, the word for created is *Bārā;* it means to create, form, make, produce, bring into existence. Bārā emphasizes the initiation of the object, not manipulating it after original creation. It refers only to an activity, which can be performed by God. Therefore; In the beginning, God created, formed, produced, brought into existence the heavens and the earth from nothing. John 1:3 says, all things came into being through Him; and apart from Him, nothing came into being that has come into being.

The earth was formless and void, and darkness was over the surface of the deep, and the Spirit of God was moving over the surface of the waters.
(Genesis 1:2)

In Genesis 1:2, the earth was described as formless, void, and dark, but the Spirit of God was present. He moved over the surface of the waters. The analogy of "moved over the surface of the water" is like a fowl continually brooding over hatching eggs. God had a plan and purpose for the earth and when God is present, things just can't remain the same.

Then God said, "Let there be light," and there was light. God saw that the light was good, and God separated the light from the darkness. God called the light day, and the darkness He called night. And there was evening and there was morning, one day

Genesis 1:3-5

When God spoke, there was an immediate result. When He said, "let there be light," at His command, light appeared. He saw that the light was good and separated light from darkness. Day and night were established. Many times, when we think about night and day, we think about the sun creating light and night is when the sun goes down and the moon rises. Yet at this particular time, the sun and moon have yet to be created. On the first day of creation, there is a separation of light and darkness. I find it interesting that the separation of light and darkness is one of God's first recorded actions. We see him still performing this action today with his people:

For you are all sons of light and sons of day. We are not of night nor of darkness 1 Thessalonians 5:5 (NASB95)

I have come as Light into the world, so that everyone who believes in Me will not remain in darkness John 12:46

You may be asking how is this relevant to my health? How can this be beneficial to me during a pandemic? One example of the relevance of day and night is that scientists found small nuclei in the hypothalamus of the brain called the suprachiasmatic nucleus (SCN). These nuclei are responsible for controlling the circadian rhythms of all living organisms: bacteria, plants, fungi, animals, and humans. Franz Halberg introduced the concept of the circadian rhythm in 1959. The circadian rhythm was found to function in a 24-hour cycle and respond to light and darkness. The circadian rhythm influences the sleep wake cycle, body temperature, hormone secretion, cell division and proliferation, gastro-intestinal tract function, reproductive function, metabolism, and body mass regulation. The pineal gland secrets 80% of the melatonin produced in our body and the majority of melatonin is made during the night. Melatonin promotes sleep, while cortisol is produced during the day, so we can stay awake. Melatonin is released optimally in total darkness after you have been asleep 3 to 5 hours. Sleep deprivation decreases the immune system.

Recent studies have shown that melatonin has an effect on the Coronavirus

Melatonin, known as the hormone of darkness, is one of my favorite hormones. Melatonin has many wonderful properties beyond getting a good night's sleep. It controls the sleep wake cycle; it is a powerful antioxidant, it is responsible for maintaining homeostasis; it is an anxiolytic, and upregulates glutathione. It has been successfully used to treat delirium, atherosclerosis, respiratory disease, and viral infections. It also suppresses NF-KB, an inflammatory process. When melatonin is combined with vitamin C, E and glutathione, it has a markedly enhanced protective effect on removing free radicals from the body. Free radicals can cause damage to cells, protein and DNA.

Studies showed that melatonin's antioxidative, anti-inflammatory, and immune-enhancing properties can help protect against acute lung injury (ALI) and acute respiratory distress syndrome (ARDS). When a person is infected with the Coronavirus, the virus attaches to receptors found in the lungs. When the virus attaches itself to the receptors, it replicates and causes damage to lung tissue and possibly leads to ALI and ARDS. According to the study (COVID-19, pneumonia

& inflammasomes—the melatonin connection), it is believed that regardless of age, if a person has adequate amounts of melatonin, the infectiousness of COVID-19 will be greatly reduced, and the chances of developing ARD or ALI is significantly diminished.

Melatonin production:

- Melatonin is produced from protein, therefore, it is necessary that we have adequate protein intake to make melatonin.
- Vitamin B5, B6, iron, zinc, and SAMe are needed to convert protein into melatonin. If we are deficient in these nutrients, melatonin production will be compromised.

- When the sun begins to go down, and it begins to get dark, the suprachiasmatic nucleus (SCN) signals the pineal gland to release melatonin. Melatonin is only released from the pineal gland when it is dark.

Helpful hints so your body can make adequate amounts of melatonin

- Avoid looking at electronic devices or TV screens at least two hours before bedtime, or use glasses that can block out blue light (blue light blocking glasses)
- Sleep in total darkness- covering lights from TV, DVD/Blue-ray players, windows, alarm clocks, etc. Light reduces melatonin production

- Use red lights for night lights-
  red light has the least power
  to shift the circadian rhythm
  and suppress melatonin
- Don't check cell phone
  messages in the middle of the
  night
- If you have to have the TV on
  to go to sleep, set the timer to
  cut off in 30 minutes
- Night shift workers-wear
  glasses that block out blue
  light

Most people are familiar with the
supplement, melatonin, and may
take it if they have trouble sleeping
or to help with jet lag when flying to
different time zones. I can attest to
the fact that melatonin helps with
jet lag. I take it when traveling to
different time zones to help
acclimate my body to the time
change. Melatonin has also been
found in plants. The root, leaves,
and fruit of plants contain

melatonin. Certain plants have higher concentrations than others. For example, banana, pineapple, citrus fruit, tart sour cherries, walnuts, corn, rice and peanuts have significant amounts of melatonin. Eating these foods can help increase melatonin, the healing hormone in your body.

Supplementing with melatonin

Safety/ Side effects

- Safe for long-term use
- Studies show it's safe at 300mg/day for 2 years
- Not to be taken by children under 9 years old, as they make high levels of melatonin
- Take at night—1-2 hours before bedtime, 2-3 hours after last meal
- Minor side effects experienced by some patients: lethargy, headache,

rash, upset stomach, sleep disorders, vivid dreams
- Some studies show that melatonin is beneficial; others show it is contraindicated in: glucose intolerance, seizures, Multiple sclerosis, and autoimmune diseases.

Recommendation (information from the COVID-19, pneumonia & melatonin connection study)

Maintenance dosages:
.2-.5mg- at night

COVID-19 positive
5-50mg/day
- Lower dosage for younger age and no or mild symptoms.
- Higher dosage for older age and moderate to severe symptoms.

During an active infection: 40% of the daily dose should be divided into small portions and taken every 2hrs during the day. 60% of the total dose should be divided into 2 portions and taken 2-3hours after dinner. The final dose should be completed by 10 pm.

Supplements

Melatonin .5mg (Pure encapsulations)
https://wellevate.me/vanessa-edwards

Melaton-5 (Thorne)
https://wellevate.me/vanessa-edwards

Blue light blocking glasses (Amazon)

DIY At Home Melatonin Test
https://thor.ne/RAnuL

Genesis 1:6-8

*Then God said, "Let there be an
expanse in the midst of the
waters, and let it separate the
waters from the waters."*

*God made the expanse, and
separated the waters which
were below the
expanse from the waters which
were above the expanse; and it
was so. God called the expanse
heaven.*

*And there was evening and
there was morning, a second
day*

CHAPTER 10
DAY 2

Hydration / Hand Washing / Hand Sanitizer

Then God said, "Let there be an expanse in the midst of the waters, and let it separate the waters from the waters." God made the expanse, and separated the waters which were below the expanse from the waters which were above the expanse; and it was so. God called the expanse heaven. And there was evening and there was morning, a second day. (Genesis 1:6-8)

Keeping your immune system healthy and functioning at its best is important for your ability to fight viruses. Seventy percent of your immune system resides in the gut. Supporting immune health through good nutrition, proper rest, and hydration is important for fighting off infections.

Water Facts

Water is vital for all forms of life. Water protects the spinal cord, prevents blood clots, prohibits constipation, lowers blood pressure, and helps regulate body temperature. The human body is composed of approximately 60% water. The amount of water in the brain and heart is approximately 73%, the lungs 83%, skin 64%, muscles and kidneys 79%, bones 31%. We lose nearly one quart of water a day just by breathing. Think about a quart of milk; you are losing that much water on a daily basis just by breathing. Many people don't drink a quart of water a day to replace what they have lost. This does not even include the water you lose from sweating. So, please make a conscious effort to drink more water on a daily basis.

Water needed to eliminate toxins

Water is also important for the immune system. The body needs water for proper digestion, to carry nutrients in and out of cells, and for the removal of toxins. A healthy immune system is dependent upon proper nutrients. We will discuss this in further detail in the next chapter. In this chapter, we will focus on the role of the liver in eliminating toxins.

The liver uses vitamins and minerals to take toxins that have accumulated in the body from a toxic state to a nontoxic state using phase 1 and phase 2 of liver detoxification. Once the toxins are broken down, they are transformed into a water-soluble state, so that they can be removed from the body via the kidneys or the bowel. This process can be inhibited if you are dehydrated. Therefore, toxins will remain in the body and suppress the immune system. When the immune system is suppressed, the ability of the immune system to recognize and eliminate foreign invaders like bacteria and viruses is compromised.

How do you know if you are dehydrated?

According to MayoClinic, symptoms of mild to moderate dehydration can be feeling thirsty. Therefore, when you have the sensation of thirst, you are already in a state of mild to moderate dehydration. Other symptoms include dry mouth, decreased urine output, dry skin, few or no tears when crying, headache, constipation, dizziness, lightheadedness, and edema. You may be surprised by the fact that dehydration can cause edema; the body is actually trying to retain as much fluid as possible. Severe dehydration can be a medical emergency. Symptoms of severe dehydration include extreme thirst, irritability, confusion, very dry mouth, little or no urination, sunken eyes, dry skin that lacks elasticity and doesn't "bounce back" when pinched, low blood pressure, rapid heartbeat, rapid breathing, no tears when crying, and fever. The color of urine can also be an indicator. Clear or light-colored urine indicates hydration, while dark yellow or amber-colored urine indicates dehydration.

How much water should we drink?

For years, we have heard that we should drink eight glasses of water a day. Recent studies have shown that drinking half your body weight in ounces per day is more accurate. To calculate this, divide your weight by two—this is how much water in ounces you need on a daily basis. For example, a person who weighs 100 pounds needs 50oz of water daily.

I don't like the taste of water, what can I do?

Add a slice of organic lemon, lime, or orange to add flavor and electrolytes to your water. You can also enhance the flavor of water by adding organic cinnamon sticks, peppermint, or spearmint leaves.

Dangers of sugary drinks

I do realize that on the third day, God separated the waters. But I just can't leave this chapter without addressing the many sugary drinks we consume, and how it affects us physically. Most 12oz cans of soda contain 9-10 teaspoons or more of sugar. The World Health Organization (WHO) has set the recommended daily allowance of sugar to be no more than 6 teaspoons a day, which is 25 grams. The USDA sets the maximum amount of sugar at 10 teaspoons per day. Yet, the body only needs 4/5 tsp—4 grams—of sugar to maintain healthy glucose levels. Let's take a look at the sugar content of some popular soft drinks. Coca Cola has 39 grams; Mountain Dew, 46 grams, and Pepsi has 41 grams of sugar. Now, let's take a look at fruit juices. Many times, juice is substituted for soda because you are trying to make healthier choices. Yet, juices made from concentrate can have more or just as much sugar as soda. For example, twelve ounces of grape juice has 58g of sugar, apple juice has 39 grams of sugar, and orange juice has 33 grams of sugar. We oftentimes give kids boxed juices. They are convenient, but most are not 100 percent juice. They contain added sugar, coloring, and flavoring. If juice is made from a concentrated source, it has higher levels of sugar—many contain high fructose corn syrup and/or artificial sweeteners. Please be aware of what your kids drink; it makes a difference. Please read labels.

What happens physiologically when soda is consumed?

When a can of soda is consumed, blood sugar levels spike within 20 minutes. In response to this elevated blood sugar level, the pancreas releases insulin. This insulin in turn tries to get glucose (sugar) inside the cell. After approximately 40 minutes, the cells have absorbed caffeine, which causes blood pressure to rise. After 45 minutes, dopamine, a neurotransmitter in the brain, is increased and stimulates the reward and pleasure part of the brain, giving a heroin drug-like feelings. This leads to addiction. This is why it is so hard for many people to stop drinking sodas.

Obesity, Diabetes, COVID-19

Elevated sugar consumption contributes to diabetes, obesity and high blood pressure, which are all comorbidities that lead to higher death rates when infected with the Coronavirus. The incidence of diabetes rose from 5.6 million in 1980 to 20.9 million in 2011.

According to the CDC, drinking one or two cans of sugary drinks a day increases the risk of type 2 diabetes by 26%. Obesity affects 78.6 million adults and 12.7 million children and adolescents in America. One report showed that 85% of obese individuals that tested positive for the Coronavirus had to be put on ventilators compared to 47% of infected healthy weight individuals that tested positive for the virus. In New York City, out of the 5,279 patients that tested positive for the Coronavirus between March 1 and April 8 2020, 22% were diabetic and 35.3% were obese. In Britain, those who suffered from obesity were twice as likely to develop severe complications from COVID-19.

Water for washing hands

Wash your hands with soap and water. You have heard this over and over again. It is a simple yet highly effective habit to have. It is not necessary to purchase antibacterial soap. Studies show that there is no evidence that antibacterial soap works any better than soap without these chemicals. Actually, many chemicals in antibacterial soaps were banned because they were found to be harmful.

What's the most effective way to wash your hands?

Use warm water and soap. Rubbing hands together, making sure you cover every surface of your hands: palms, back of hands, in between fingers, and don't forget your fingernails. Wash for 20 seconds, then rinse. Dry using a single-use towel or air dry.

When should I wash my hands?

- After touching surfaces others might have touched— such as door handles, elevator buttons, railings, computers, phone, mouse, self-check-out, etc.
- After touching your mask- while removing, applying, or adjusting
- After you cough, sneeze, or blow your nose. (It is better to cover a cough or sneeze in the crease of your elbow)
- Before preparing food
- Before eating
- After eating
- After you use the restroom

What should I do when soap and water is not available?

When soap and water are not available, hand sanitizer can be used. It's convenient and has the ability to kill viruses. Hand sanitizer should contain at least 60% ethanol or 70% isopropanol. Lesser strengths will not have an effect on viruses. It is important that you read labels when choosing hand sanitizer.

What ingredients should not be in hand sanitizer?

Hand sanitizers should not contain methanol, fragrance, or parfum.

Methanol has been in the news recently. Some companies are using methanol or wood alcohol as a substitute for ethanol or isopropyl alcohol. Methanol has many side effects such as nausea, vomiting, headache, blurred vision, permanent blindness, seizures, coma, permanent damage to the nervous system and even death.

Fragrance or parfum is in the category of chemicals called phthalates. These chemicals, found in many hand sanitizers, have not made the news yet are something we need to be aware of. According to the CDC, phthalates are a group of chemicals used to make plastics more flexible and harder to break. They are also used as solvents or dissolving agents for other materials. They are found in many personal care products such as soap, shampoo, hair spray, nail polish, and hand sanitizer. Side effects listed on the environmental working groups website, include: adverse effects on human reproduction and development, reproductive system birth defects in baby boys. Phthalates are endocrine (hormone) disrupters, which can possibly cause cancer. I know you are very engaged in this book right now, but if you could just stop reading for a few minutes, look at your personal care products and hand sanitizers to see if they have any of the ingredients listed above. Please be aware and beware!

Genesis 1:11-13

Then God said, "Let the earth sprout vegetation, plants yielding seed, and fruit trees on the earth bearing fruit after their kind with seed in ;" and it was so.

The earth brought forth vegetation, plants yielding seed after their kind, and trees bearing fruit with seed in them, after their kind; and God saw that it was good.

There was evening and there was morning, the third day.

CHAPTER 11
Day 3

Vitamins / Minerals / The Immune System

Then God said, "Let the earth sprout vegetation, plants yielding seed, and fruit trees on the earth bearing fruit after their kind with seed in them;" and it was so. The earth brought forth vegetation, plants yielding seed after their kind, and trees bearing fruit with seed in them, after their kind; and God saw that it was good. There was evening and there was morning, the third day. (Genesis 1:11-13)

Elohim, God, our creator spoke and the earth began to sprout forth vegetables, herbs, fruit, grains, nuts, and seeds. On the third day, God provided nutrients, vitamins, minerals, enzymes, fiber, and antioxidants. He provided the fuel needed for the body to operate optimally. We were provided with the nutrients necessary for the body to heal itself and to sustain life to come. Food should be our first line of defense. Supplements do not take the place of a healthy diet; they are just what they say they are—a supplement to healthy nutrition. During a pandemic is a great time to increase certain supplements in order to arm your body with added protection from bacteria and viruses. We will take a look at a few nutrients that have the potential to help the immune system defend itself against these foreign invaders.

Vitamin C

In regards to the Coronavirus, studies have shown that vitamin C, vitamin A, zinc, and glutathione have significant roles to play in how the immune system responds to viruses. This could possibly have an impact on the severity of symptoms one experiences and how long one would experience them. We will begin by taking a look at vitamin C. Vitamin C, also known as ascorbic acid, cannot be made by the human body. We must get vitamin C from food or supplementation. Vitamin C has antioxidant, anti-inflammatory, and immune-supporting properties. The white blood cells (WBC)—the body's defense system—stores vitamin C. During an infection, vitamin C levels within the WBC's are depleted rapidly. This depletion of vitamin C can decrease the body's defense system, antioxidants, and lead to inflammation. When vitamin C levels are maintained during an infection, this allows the defense system to stay armed and inflammation is kept in check. Vitamin C has been shown to support respiratory defense mechanisms, prevent viral infections, and reduce the duration and severity of an infection. Vitamin C also has antihistamine properties that can improve flu-like symptoms. In the study, *the clinical effects of vitamin C supplementation in elderly hospitalized patients with acute respiratory infections* results showed that vitamin C administration reduced the severity and duration of pneumonia in elderly patients. As you know, the elderly are being affected by the virus at higher rates and many are not recovering. Could something as simple as supplementing with vitamin C help save lives?

The article, *micronutrient status of COVID-19 patients: a critical consideration,* addresses how little attention is paid to the micronutrient status of COVID-19 patients. Vitamin C is a micronutrient. A micronutrient is a substance required in trace amounts for the normal growth and development of living organisms. Micronutrients consist of vitamins and minerals that play a critical role in the proper function of proteins, enzymes, and physiological processes within the body. Without micronutrients, the body cannot function properly. On a daily basis, the body only requires small amounts of micronutrients, usually micrograms, in order to function properly. But the need increases significantly when a person is ill. For example, critically ill patients were admitted to the hospital and their vitamin C levels were severely depleted and required vitamin C in grams to replete the patients. One common complication of severe vitamin C deficiency is pneumonia. Pneumonia is one of the most common causes of mortality in patients with severe vitamin C deficiency. Vitamin C status of patients with COVID-19 has not been reported in literature, but past studies have shown that the vitamin C levels of patients with community-acquired pneumonia is severely depleted and associated with enhanced oxidative stress. Physicians, knowing the micronutrient levels of their COVID-19 patients and supplementing with adequate amounts to restore normal status and function, may help improve patient outcomes.

Intravenous (IV) use of Vitamin C

There is a pressing need for safe, effective, and inexpensive therapies that can alter the natural course of the disease process of COVID-19 and reduce the strain on healthcare systems. High dose intravenous (IV) vitamin C has been shown to be safe and effective in acute respiratory distress syndrome (ARDS) from viral origins. A double-blind, placebo controlled randomized clinical trial involving 167 patients with ARDS was performed. Patients suffering from ARDS were given IV vitamin C every 6 hours for 4 days or a regular standard of care with placebo. The results were significant; only 29.8% in the group receiving vitamin C died, compared to 46.3% deaths in the placebo group.

Many physicians in Shanghai, China, utilize IV vitamin C in the treatment of COVID-19. Dr. Richard Z. Cheng, a Chinese-American specialist physician, who works closely with the medical and governmental authorities throughout China, has been instrumental in encouraging hospitals to implement vitamin C therapy. He has also been involved in facilitating several clinical trials using IV vitamin C that are currently underway. Dr. Cheng also recommends supplementing with vitamin C to prevent COVID-19. On March 3, 2020, the government of Shanghai, China, announced an official recommendation that COVID-19 should be treated with IV vitamin C.

Below is an official statement from Xi'an Jiaotong University Second Hospital:

"On the afternoon of February 20, 2020, another 4 patients with severe new coronaviral pneumonia recovered from the C10 West Ward of Tongji Hospital. In the past, 8

patients have been discharged from this hospital. High-dose vitamin C achieved good results in clinical applications. We believe that for patients with severe neonatal pneumonia and critically ill patients, vitamin C treatment should be initiated as soon as possible after admission. Early application of large doses of vitamin C can have a strong antioxidant effect, reduce inflammatory responses, and improve endothelial function. Numerous studies have shown that the dose of vitamin C has a lot to do with the effect of treatment. High-dose vitamin C can not only improve antiviral levels but more importantly, can prevent and treat acute lung injury (ALI) and acute respiratory distress (ARDS)."

Foods High in Vitamin C

- Red / Green peppers-raw
- Kiwi
- Chili peppers
- Broccoli (cooked/raw)
- Strawberries
- Brussels sprouts (cooked)
- Kale
- Pineapple
- Mango
- cauliflower

Recommendations (information from the COVID-19, pneumonia & melatonin connection study)

COVID-19 positive

1gram every 15 - 30min, depending on the severity of symptoms.

Increase to 2 grams every 15-30min, if symptoms not reversed within 12-24hrs

Maintenance

Liposomal vitamin C: 1 squirt hold in mouth 30 seconds then swallow, 3 times daily.
Buffered vitamin C: ½ scoop in water, 2 times daily.

Liposomal vitamin C (Seeking Health)
https://wellevate.me/vanessa-edwards

Buffered vitamin C (Thorne)
https://wellevate.me/vanessa-edwards

Vitamin A

Like vitamin C, vitamin A is an essential micronutrient that can not be manufactured by the human body. We must supply the body with this nutrient from our diet and through supplementation. Once consumed, vitamin A is stored in the liver until it is needed. Vitamin A is found in two forms, retinol and carotenoids. Retinol is the active form of vitamin A found in animal liver, whole milk, and some fortified foods. Carotenoids are found in plant foods that can turn into the active form of vitamin A. There are over 500 known carotenoids. A very familiar one is beta-carotene. Beta-carotene is an antioxidant. Antioxidants protect cells from damage caused by free radicals. Vitamin A plays a role in having good eyesight, a strong skeletal system, daily replacement of skin cells, and helping to maintain a healthy immune system. We will focus on vitamin A's ability to maintain a healthy immune system.

Vitamin A deficiency COVID-19

In order for the immune system to function properly, it is dependent upon vitamin A. Vitamin A is responsible for the maturation of white blood cells (WBC) called neutrophils. Neutrophils are the most abundant type of WBC in the body and are considered the first responders of the defense system. When the body encounters foreign bacteria or viruses, the demand for vitamin A increases and the defense system goes into action. The body increases the number of neutrophils that are in the bloodstream; the neutrophils recognize and kill unwanted bacteria. The neutrophils literally engulf the bacteria like Pac man engulfed the dots. When the bacteria are engulfed, toxins are released inside the cell and the bacteria are killed; game over. When a person is experiencing vitamin A deficiency, their neutrophil count will increase when they encounter bacteria, but the ability of the WBC to kill bacteria is impaired. Therefore, when neutrophils engulf bacteria and there is not enough vitamin A on board, the WBC's die and the bacteria continue to proliferate. This impairment can cause the body to be vulnerable and susceptible to severe infections. Many patients that have COVID-19 are not only infected by the Coronavirus but will also experience secondary bacterial infections, which can lead to pneumonia. Optimal levels of vitamin A may prevent a person that has contracted the Coronavirus from worsening the disease leading to pneumonia. It may also decrease the progression of pneumonia, which can be a fatal symptom of COVID-19.

A randomized control trial consisting of 3021 children concluded that Vitamin A supplementation helps relieve clinical symptoms and signs of pneumonia and shorten the length of time the children were in the hospital.

Another study looking at Vitamin A deficiency was done on mice. This study showed that when the mice were deficient in vitamin A, there was a breakdown of the gut barrier. The gut barrier is important in keeping pathogens out of the body. When there is an impairment, this can lead to the entry of viruses into the body. Remember, as stated in chapter 7, the intestines have ACE2 receptors that the Coronavirus attaches to and enters the cells. It has been hypothesized that if vitamin A levels are optimal, the gut barrier will be intact and possibly prevent the entry of the virus.

Foods that contain vitamin A

- Carrots
- Dark green leafy vegetables
- Eggs
- Liver
- Mango
- Milk
- Papaya
- Pumpkin
- Sweet potatoes
- Squash

Recommendations
Vitamin A drops (Seeking Health)
https://wellevate.me/vanessa-edwards

Zinc

Zinc is a trace mineral found in the body and is involved in many biological processes. Zinc has been shown to support the immune system by aiding the body in producing antibodies in response to viral infections. Zinc plays a vital role in how the immune system responds to viral infections. Zinc is purported to be a vital mineral during COVID-19 infection because it has a dual responsibility. First, it has antiviral properties. The antiviral properties that zinc exhibits are its ability to inhibit the enzyme required for RNA viruses, like the coronaviruses, to replicate. Second, it acts as an immunomodulator. An immunomodulator is an agent that modifies the immune response or the functioning of the immune system by stimulating the release of antibodies or by inhibiting white blood cell activity. In layman's terms, zinc has the ability to cause the body not to over-respond to infectious agents like viruses.

People with zinc deficiency have been shown to have increased susceptibility to bacterial, viral, and fungal infections. This is because when you are deficient in zinc, this causes markers in the body that cause inflammation to increase. These markers are called pro-inflammatory cytokines: IL-1, IL-6, and TNF alpha. When there is an increase in these cytokines and there is nothing to calm them down, it can lead to organ damage; this is referred to as the cytokine storm. In the case of COVID-19, lungs are damaged due to the cytokine storm and if not gotten under control, ventilation will be required and may lead to death. Currently, zinc is being investigated for preventative treatment of patients with COVID-19.

In several studies, zinc has been shown to reduce the common cold duration and decrease mortality rates when given to adults with severe pneumonia. Zinc also reduced the incidence and prevalence of pneumonia in children.

Six randomized control trials that included 2,216 patients with severe pneumonia were given zinc as an adjunct therapy. The results showed that there was a decrease in mortality rate among those who received zinc compared to those who didn't.

Elderly deficient in zinc

As discussed previously, the Coronavirus affects older adults at a higher rate than younger adults. It has been found that many elderly patients are deficient in zinc. In a study, elderly patients in nursing homes were given 30 milligrams of zinc daily. After a period of time, results showed that zinc supplementation improved their immune system.

Zinc deficiency symptoms:

Loss of taste
Loss of smell
Hair loss
Skin rashes
Lethargy

Foods high in zinc

Oysters
Pumpkin seeds
Hemp seeds
Grass-fed beef
Chickpeas
Lentils
Cocoa powder

Cashews
Ricotta cheese
Mushrooms
Beef
Spinach
Avocado
Chicken
Almonds
Seeds
Oats

Recommendations
Biomins (Thorne)
https://wellevate.me/vanessa-edwards

Glutathione

Glutathione is an antioxidant that is made up of three amino acids: cysteine, glycine, and glutamic acid. Glutathione is the most abundant antioxidant in the body. It is found in most cells in the body. Antioxidants protect the body against oxidative or free radical damage. Free radicals can cause damage to cells and tissue. Glutathione, GSH has many important functions such as: detoxification, regeneration of vitamin C and E, neutralizing free radicals, mitochondrial health, antiviral defense, regulating immune response, and promoting longevity.

You may be asking, what is an antioxidant? Why are antioxidants so important? I will explain this by using an example from one of my favorite naturopathic doctors, Dr. Ben Lynch. He explains oxidation this way, in his book, Dirty Genes. Our bodies burn oxygen for fuel, which is a good thing, but that process produces various harmful chemicals and by-products such as hydrogen peroxide and free radicals. In order to protect cells from these harmful chemicals and by-products, the cells need a lot of glutathione. He describes glutathione as the "primary protector."

When a person is infected with the Coronavirus, the body responds by releasing pro-inflammatory chemicals such as cytokines and chemokines to help kill the virus. The virus has several protective mechanisms that help it to continue to replicate, disregarding the bodies mounting attack against it. This mounted attack leads to inflammation and the production of reactive oxygen species, (ROS)-oxidative stress. When this response occurs, glutathione, the primary protector, comes to the rescue. The longer the symptoms persist, the more glutathione is needed. If glutathione is not replenished, it will be depleted.

In a very small study, glutathione and ROS levels were tested in four females that tested positive for COVID-19. The females were all nonsmokers and free from chronic disease. Two of the ladies only experienced mild symptoms: both had a mild fever, one had mild muscle aches, and the other had mild fatigue. Their symptoms were gone within 4-6 days. They both had optimal levels of glutathione, .712/.933, and low levels of ROS, 2.07/1.143. The third female in the study experienced moderate to severe symptoms, which included: fever, dry cough, shortness of breath, significant fatigue, and increase heart rate. Her symptoms were relieved in 16 days. Her glutathione levels were .531 and ROS levels were high, 3.677. The fourth patient experienced severe symptoms: fever, dry cough, hoarseness, significant muscle pain, fatigue and pneumonia. Twenty-four days later, the symptoms still persisted. Her glutathione levels were very low, 0.079, and the ROS levels were elevated at 2.73. It can be hypothesized that glutathione deficiency can lead to serious side effects, being manifested due to COVID-19. This study stated that "since the antiviral effect of glutathione is nonspecific, there is reason to believe that glutathione is also active against SARS- CoV-2. Therefore, restoration of glutathione levels in COVID-19 patients would be a promising

approach for the management of
the novel coronavirus SARS-CoV-2."

NAC-precursor to glutathione

N-Acetylcysteine (NAC) is a
precursor to glutathione. When you
supply your body with NAC, it will
breakdown into glutathione. Long-
term oral administration of NAC has
been tested and has been found to
have preventive properties against
respiratory viral infections. NAC is
widely available, safe, and
reasonably priced. It is very difficult
to find a quality glutathione
supplement that is actually
absorbable. There are only a couple
on the market that I would suggest.
They can be found in the
recommendation section below.

Ways to raise glutathione levels

Eat fruits and vegetables

Eat organic when possible
Eat almonds
NAC
Vitamin C
Meditation (meditating on God's word raises levels by 20%)
Good night's sleep
Decrease toxic exposure

Things that deplete glutathione

Stress
Carbohydrates
Foods high in sugar
Infections: bacterial or viral
Alcohol
Smoking
Mold
Yeast
Parasites
Chemicals

Foods that increase glutathione

Spinach
Avocado
Asparagus
Okra
Fish
Chicken
Beef
Broccoli
Brussel sprouts
Cauliflower
Kale
Mustard greens
Watercress
Garlic
Onions
Shallots
Turmeric
Curcumin

Recommendations

NAC (Seeking Health)
https://wellevate.me/vanessa-edwards

Optimal Liposomal Glutathione Plus
(Seeking Health)
https://wellevate.me/vanessa-edwards

Optimal Liposomal Glutathione
(Seeking Health)
https://wellevate.me/vanessa-edwards

Safe Cell (Tesseract)
www.DSSOrders.com/DrEdwards
Registration Code   VE1366

Curcumin

Curcumin is the predominant curcuminoid found in turmeric. Curcumin has had positive reviews in regulating the immune response with influenza A, by helping to prevent lung injury. Curcumin has antiviral, anti-inflammatory, antimicrobial, and antioxidant properties. It also has the ability to reduce cytokine production. Therefore, it may be a great choice to help prevent lung injury from COVID-19. As to date, there have not been any research studies published with patients positive for COVID-19 using Curcumin, also known as turmeric. Curcumin is safe. It has been used as a spice for centuries. I recommend Meriva, Meriva pairs curcumin with a phytosome for a 29x greater absorption rate than other curcumins on the market. Meriva is the most clinically studied curcumin and has been found to also help with joint support, liver detoxification, and GI support.

Foods
Tumeric root/powder
Curry powder

Recommendations
Meriva (Thorne)
https://thor.ne/Vlt1a

Genesis 1:14-19

*Then God said, "Let there be lights in
the expanse of the heavens to
separate the day from the night, and
let them be for signs and for seasons
and for days and years; and let them
be for lights in the expanse of the
heavens to give light on the earth;"
and it was so. God made the two
great lights, the greater light to
govern the day, and the lesser light
to govern the night; He made the
stars also. God placed them in the
expanse of the heavens to give light
on the earth, and to govern the day
and the night, and to separate the
light from the darkness; and God saw
that it was good. There was evening
and there was morning, the fourth
day.*

CHAPTER 12
Day 4

The "Sunshine" Vitamin

On the fourth day, God appointed the Sun to govern the day and the moon to govern the night. He placed them in the heavens to give light to the earth. Are there other benefits to the sun other than giving light to the earth? Yes, God tends to do more than one thing at a time. Sun exposure happens to be the main source of Vitamin D for humans. Today, we tend to hear more about the risks associated with sun exposure and less about the benefits. There are many warnings about getting too much sun. I don't want to down play this because overexposure can lead to basal cell and squamous cell carcinoma, skin cancer. It is estimated that 3.5 million people are diagnosed with skin cancer each year in the United States. Yet, there are many benefits to sun exposure. Direct sunlight is very important in creating vitamin D3 (cholecalciferol). The predominant source of vitamin D3 is formed by ultraviolet B rays from the sun, making direct contact with the skin. This means you can't make vitamin D while you are in your car, enjoying the warmth of the sunlight with the windows rolled up and the air conditioner blasting. The rays from the sun must come in direct contact with the skin. Only about 20% of vitamin D is found in dietary sources. Foods that contain vitamin D naturally are wild caught salmon, tuna, mackerel, sardines, alfalfa sprouts, mushrooms, and eggs. Since many Americans don't eat a lot of these foods on a daily basis, foods such as milk, orange juice, and cereal were fortified with vitamin D in the 1930's to try to make up for the deficiency. The problem with fortification is that vitamin D is not very heat-stable; therefore, 10-50% may be degraded with heat.

Vitamin D deficiency is a global problem. We are spending more time indoors than outside, soaking up those ultraviolet B rays. Nursing homes have been hit hard by the Coronavirus. Could this be related to a lack of vitamin D? When a person is in the nursing home, the amount of sun that they are exposed to is very little or none at all. At the beginning of the pandemic, we were ordered to stay at home or to quarantine, in an attempt to get the virus under control. While I think there is a place for quarantine, I believe it is just part of the solution. During the stay at home order, we should have been encouraged to go outside and to take vitamin D supplements. Instead, when reporters asked medical professionals, should vitamin D be taken or if it played a role in the pandemic, we were told that vitamin D could not help with this pandemic. This really upset me. Just think, if we had spent a month fortifying our bodies with nutrients, including vitamin D, and then went back out into the community, this could have decreased the spread of the virus and saved lives.

Stay at home order in the United Kingdom

In June 2020, when the residents of the United Kingdom were given the stay at home order, they were also encouraged to take 400iu's of vitamin D daily. Vitamin D was recommended because the residents would have less contact with the sun due to the stay at home order. As of September, the UK has had a total of 404,000 COVID-19 cases and 41,825 deaths, as compared to the United States of America total cases of 6.8 million over 200,000 deaths.

Vitamin D

Vitamin D is a vitamin that requires fat to be absorbed (fat-soluble), and it is also a prohormone. There are two types of vitamin D, D2 (ergocalciferol) and, D3 (cholecalciferol). Cholecalciferol (vitamin D3) occurs naturally in the body. It is synthesized when the skin is exposed to direct ultraviolet B radiation (UVB) from the sun and from the diet. Vitamin D is metabolized by the liver to 25(OH)D or 25-hydroxyvitamin D, then converted by the kidneys into 1,25-dihydroxyvitamin D or the active form of vitamin D. Vitamin D has many functions, including promoting normal bone formation and mineralization by causing calcium and phosphate to be absorbed by the intestine. It also has the ability to modulate the immune system.

Factors that inhibit vitamin D production

Location: History confirms that humans were created near the equator in Africa, where there is plenty of direct sunshine most of the year. This enabled them to produce thousands of IU's (international units) of vitamin D daily. The darker pigmentation protected them from sun-induced damage. As migration to areas with less sun, farther away from the equator, skin pigmentation became less, skin tones became lighter in order for vitamin D to be produced with less direct sunlight. Our ancestors spent many hours outside, year-round. However, this has changed drastically. We spend most of our time indoors or in cars, which shields us from direct sun exposure. Or when we do spend time outdoors, sunscreen is used. This blocks the production of vitamin D. The number of people who died from COVID-19 was lower in countries that are closer to the equator. This suggests that vitamin D may play a role in COVID-19.

A study was done on two groups of students attending osteopathic medical school. The study consisted of 359 students at two different campuses. One campus was located in sunny Florida, while the other campus was located in Pennsylvania. The study was trying to see if latitude had an effect on vitamin D levels. The results showed that only 5% of those living in Florida were deficient in vitamin D compared to a 13% deficiency in those residing in Pennsylvania.

Season: Those who live north of the equator will have a very difficult time making vitamin D during the winter months, November to March. During this time of the year, the earth is rotated away from the sun and more ultraviolet B rays are absorbed by the ozone layer, decreasing the UVB rays that make direct contact with the skin. The coronavirus outbreak is following the same pattern as the influenza virus. The virus peaks during the winter months. I believe this is due to decreased sun exposure, leading to vitamin D deficiency.

Time of day: Vitamin D production is highest between the hours of 10 a.m. and 3 p.m. because the sun's UVB rays are strongest during this time. Studies show that a minimum of 5-10 minutes of direct sunlight without sunscreen is needed in order to produce a sufficient amount of vitamin D. However, this time frame will have to be modified for people with darker skin tones. Those with darker skin tones require at least three to five times longer exposure in direct sun in order to make the same amount of vitamin D as people with white skin tones. Another obstacle to making adequate amounts of vitamin D is location. Those who live farther away from the equator will be exposed to less UVB rays; therefore more time is needed to make adequate amounts of vitamin D. There is a great app that can be downloaded for free, called Dminder. You input your location and vitamin D level; it will determine the best time of day and length of time you need to be outside to soak in vitamin D.

Darker skin tone: People with darker complexions have higher amounts of melanin or pigment in their skin. Higher melanin content reduces the skin's ability to produce vitamin D from sun exposure. Those with darker skin tones require at least three to five times longer exposure in direct sun in order to make the same amount of vitamin D as people with white skin tones.

Age: The skin's ability to synthesize vitamin D declines as we get older. Older adults are also less likely to spend a lot of time outdoors. Yet, age does not have an effect on vitamin D levels being raised with supplementation.

Polluted areas: Residents of urban areas are twice as likely to have vitamin D deficiency than people who live in rural areas. This is related to an increase in air pollution in urban areas. Air pollution hinders ultraviolet B rays, which are needed to produce vitamin D from direct contact with the skin, from reaching the earth's surface.

Pharmaceutical drugs that inhibit vitamin D production

Some medications can lead to vitamin D deficiency:

- Orlistat- weight-loss drug can lead to reduced vitamin D absorption
- Statin drugs- (Lovastatin, Simvastatin, Lipitor) reduce vitamin D production

- Cholestyramine- reduces vitamin D production
- Antiepileptic medication
- Steroids-(Prednisone, Deltasone, Rayos, Sterapred) can impair vitamin D metabolism.

In the NHANES 2001-2006 survey, vitamin D deficiency was more than twice as common among children and adults who reported oral steroid use compared to non-oral steroid users

Medical conditions that decrease vitamin D absorption

- Celiac's disease
- Chron's disease

- Kidney disease
- Liver disease
- Cystic fibrosis
- Low magnesium
- Low vitamin K
- Gastric bypass surgery
- Breastfed infants whose moms are vitamin D deficient
- Obesity

Vitamin D / COVID-19

Studies show that vitamin D may be useful in decreasing the risk of COVID-19. The mechanisms used by vitamin D are: its ability to lower viral replication, increase anti-inflammatory cytokines, and reduce pro-inflammatory cytokines. When pro-inflammatory cytokines are produced, there is a decrease in anti-inflammatory cytokines. This leads to an inflammation process that can cause damage to lung tissue and lead to pneumonia. If this inflammation process progresses, it could lead to a hyper response of the immune system known as the cytokine storm. Vitamin D may have the ability to prevent viral replication if exposed and possibly prevent this overreaction of the immune system to the Coronavirus.

The Research:

In the fall and winter of 2009-2010, an observational study was conducted in Connecticut. They looked at 198 healthy adults and examined the relationship between their vitamin D levels and the incidence of them having acute respiratory tract infections. Results showed that only 17% of those who maintained vitamin D levels greater than 38ng/ml throughout the study developed acute respiratory tract infections, while 45% of those who had levels lower than 38 ng/ml developed acute respiratory tract infections.

A review of eleven randomized control trials consisting of 5,660 participants found that vitamin D decreased the risk of respiratory infections.

This next study is a study that was published by the University of Chicago. I personally believe this study should have made local and international news. If implemented, these results can be beneficial to so many people.

On September 3, 2020, JAMA published a study that showed an association between low vitamin D status and positive COVID-19 test results. The study consisted of 489 patients who had a vitamin D test in the year prior to the pandemic. The average age of the participants was 49.2 years old; the study consisted of mostly females (75%), and there was a large representation of people of color. Blacks/ African Americans, Asians/ Mideast Indians, and those who reported multiple race made up 68% of the study. Vitamin D deficiency was found in 172 participants. In this study, vitamin D deficiency was defined as those with vitamin D, 25-hydroxycholecalciferol levels less than 20ng/ml. Thirty-two out of the 172 participants with vitamin D levels less than 20 tested positive for COVID-19. Only 39 participants tested positive out of the 317 participants whose levels were higher than 20ng/ml. This is great news. This study shows that when your vitamin D levels are deficient, you have a greater chance of contracting COVID-19, but the opposite is true as well. When your vitamin D levels are higher than 20, I suggest optimal levels of vitamin D, which is 60-70ng/ml, the chances of you actually contracting the coronavirus decreases remarkably.

Miscarriages/ COVID-19/ Vitamin D deficiency

The incidence of miscarriages due to COVID-19 is rising. At the beginning of the pandemic, pregnant women were told that they were not at increased risk. As time has gone on and the number of women suffering miscarriages after having a positive COVID-19 diagnosis has increased, the CDC had to revise the COVID-19 risk during pregnancy.

Previous studies showed that when pregnant women were infected by viruses such as: SARS-CoV, H1N1, and MERS, there was an increased incidence of spontaneous abortions, premature delivery and intrauterine growth restriction. In this study, it was suggested that women take vitamin D because it has the ability to suppress viral replication and the ability to modulate the immune system. Recent studies confirm that the placenta can be infected with SARS-CoV2. After delivery, women's placentas were tested and found to be positive for coronavirus.

Data was analyzed from a study that was done to see if low dose aspirin could prevent miscarriages in women with a history of pregnancy loss. During this study, vitamin D levels were tested on 1,200 women before pregnancy and in the eighth week of pregnancy. Vitamin D deficiency was reported as levels less than 30ng/ml. The results showed that women who had vitamin D levels higher than

30ng/ml were 10% more likely to become pregnant and 15% more likely to have a live birth, compared to those whose vitamin D levels were less than 30ng/ml. The results also showed that as vitamin D levels increased by 10ng/ml at preconception, the risk of losing the baby was lowered by 12%.

The above studies are not a guarantee that a woman pregnant with COVID-19 will not suffer a miscarriage, but it is a simple, cost-effective way to possibly prevent a miscarriage. I would highly suggest that vitamin D levels be checked and vitamin D be taken to maintain levels around 70ng/ml.

Which form of Vitamin D is more effective, D2 or D3?

Vitamin D3 also known as cholecalciferol, is metabolized in the liver as 25-hydroxyvitamin D3.

D3 is produced by direct skin contact with ultraviolet rays from the sun; it is also found in animal sources such as oily fish, fish oils, egg yolks, butter and through supplementation. Vitamin D3 is more effective at increasing blood levels than vitamin D2.

Vitamin D2, also known as ergocalciferol, is metabolized in the liver as 25-hydroxyvitamin D2. D2 is found in plant sources such as mushrooms grown in ultraviolet light, fortified foods, and dietary supplements. It is less effective than D3 at increasing vitamin D blood levels.

How much vitamin D should I take?

It is important that you get your vitamin D levels checked to know what your levels are. Your current levels will determine how much vitamin D you will need to increase your levels or keep them in an optimal range. Many make the mistake of stopping vitamin D once they get their levels into the optimal range, but dosing needs to continue in order to maintain your vitamin D levels.

There is much controversy regarding optimal vitamin D levels. The Institute of Medicine recommends levels >20ng/ml for all people. The European calcified tissue society working group defined severe vitamin D deficiency as levels less than 30nmol/L. Vitamin D levels of 30ng/ml have been recommended to minimize bone fractures. Some experts recommend a range of 40-70ng/ml. I like to see my patients in the optimal range, between 60-70ng/ml range.

Vitamin D Ranges
By Dr. Alex Vazquez

Deficient <20
Insufficient levels-20-40ng/ml
Sufficient levels 40-50ng/ml
Optimal range is 50-90ng/ml
Toxic levels >100 (rare)

**Endocrine Society of Clinical Practice
Recommended Guidelines for
maintenance doses of Vitamin D
when levels are in the optimal range**

Age	Dose
Infant-6 months	1000 IU/day
6 months-1 year	1500 IU/day
1-3 years	2,500 IU/day
4-8 years	3,000 IU/day
8 years and older	4,000 IU/day

Dosage suggestions according to the
journal of pharmacology &
pharmacotherapeutics

Treatment and prevention strategies for vitamin D supplementation

Age group	Dose if Vitamin D <30ng/ml	Maintenance Dose
0-1 year	2,000 IU/day minimum 6 weeks	400-1,000 IU/day
1-18 years	2,000 IU/day minimum 6 weeks	400-1,000 IU/day
>18	6,000 IU/day minimum 8 weeks	1,500-2,000 IU/day
Obesity, malabsorption, medications that affect absorption	6,000-10,000 IU/day	3,000-6,000 IU/day

Vitamin D Toxicity

Again, it is important that you have your vitamin D levels tested. I recently had a patient in the office who was experiencing weight loss, loss of appetite, nausea, joint pain, random nodules popping up on her hands, feet, and shoulders, elevated calcium levels, and a decrease in kidney function. I suggested she get her vitamin D levels checked; she is African American and she lives in an area that doesn't get much sun in the winter months. To my surprise, her results showed that her vitamin D level was greater than 200. I have never seen a vitamin D level that high, especially in a woman of color. She was called immediately and told to stop vitamin D supplements, an office visit was scheduled, and she was asked to bring all of her supplements and medications to the appointment. I went through all of her supplements—those prescribed by me and those she was taking on her own. Her total daily intake was over 16,000 IU's plus she had spent time outside in the sun daily for several months. While vitamin D toxicity is rare, this is a great example of why you should get your vitamin D levels tested.

Vitamin D Toxicity symptoms
Loss of appetite
Weight loss
Nausea
Joint pain
Decrease kidney function
Elevated calcium levels

Foods

Wild caught Salmon
Tuna in oil

Mackerel
Sardines
Alfalfa sprouts
Mushrooms
Egg Yolk

Recommendations
Vitamin D/K2 (Thorne)
https://thor.ne/HNt3E
Vitamin D liquid (Thorne)
https://thor.ne/LBxAW
Vitamin D3 (Seeking Health)
https://wellevate.me/vanessa-edwards

Free App- iPhone and Android-
Dminder

DIY- At Home Vitamin D Test
https://thor.ne/YO6b4

Beyond PPE: A Naturopathic Approach To COVID-19

Genesis 1:20-23

And God said, Let the waters swarm with swarms of living creatures, and let birds fly above the earth in the open firmament of heaven. And God created the great sea-monsters, and every living creature that moveth, wherewith the waters swarmed, after their kind, and every winged bird after its kind: and God saw that it was good. And God blessed them, saying, Be fruitful, and multiply, and fill the waters in the seas, and let birds multiply on the earth. And there was evening and there was morning, a fifth day.

CHAPTER 13
Day 5

Fish Oil

And God said, Let the waters swarm with swarms of living creatures, and let birds fly above the earth in the open firmament of heaven. And God created the great sea-monsters, and every living creature that moveth, wherewith the waters swarmed, after their kind, and every winged bird after its kind: and God saw that it was good. (Genesis 1:20-21)

On the fifth day, God created fish. Fish contain good fats that are necessary for human health. Fish oil or omega-3 fatty acids are essential fatty acids. They are called essential because the body does not have the ability to make them and they must be supplied through food or supplementation. There are three main omega-3 fatty acids: alpha-linolenic acid (ALA), eicosapentaenoic acid (EPA), and docosahexanoic (DHA). ALA is found in plants and EPA is found in fish. Each cell in the body has a cell wall, and it is preferable that the cell wall be comprised of omega 3 fatty acids so that the wall will be fluid to allow nutrients to enter the cell and toxins to be released from the cell. Omega 3 fatty acids are beneficial to the heart, lungs, blood vessels, endocrine system, and the immune system. EPA/DHA have anti-inflammatory properties that are able to reduce the production of cytokines that can be produced when infected with the coronavirus. When there is an abundance of cytokines released, this can lead to what is called the cytokine storm. There is a hyper-response of the immune system that creates an abundance of inflammation leading to lung damage. As previously stated, lung damage and pneumonia are classic symptoms of COVID-19. Below are a couple of studies where patients with lung diseases were given Omega 3's and improvements were seen in their health.

In April 2006, a randomized, controlled, unblinded study was published that included 100 patients that were suffering from acute lung injury and on ventilators. One group was given the standard isonitrogenous, isocaloric enteral diet, and the other group was supplemented with EPA/GLA for 14 days. Results showed that patients receiving EPA/GLA showed significant improvement in oxygenation and the length of time on the ventilator was reduced.

Another study involving 146 patients on ventilators with ARDS caused by sepsis/pneumonia, trauma, or aspiration. Patients that received EPA/GLA did better than those that just received isonitrogenous, isocaloric standard diets. Results showed that oxygen levels improved by day 4 and 7. Those receiving EPA/GLA spent less days on the ventilator and less time in intensive care. Fewer patients also experienced new organ failure damage.

What if these patients were taking fish oil prior to them getting sick or at the beginning of their illness. Could omega 3's possibly prevent illnesses from worsening?

Foods high in EPA

(Beware of farmed raised fish, can be
contaminated with mercury and
polychlorinated biphenyls-PCB's)

Wild caught salmon
Mackerel
Herring
Tuna
Halibut
Trout
Bass
Sardines
Anchovies
Blue fish
Orange roughy
Marlin

Foods high in ALA

Flaxseed/oil
Walnuts
Chia seeds

Recommendations

Omega superb (Thorne)

https://thor.ne/EEvCF

Super EPA (Thorne)

https://thor.ne/utuJH

Genesis 1:26-27

Then God said, "Let Us make man in Our image, according to Our likeness; and let them rule over the fish of the sea and over the birds of the sky and over the cattle and over all the earth, and over every creeping thing that creeps on the earth."

God created man in His own image, in the image of God He created him; male and female He created them.

CHAPTER 14
Day 6

Mind Your Microbes

Then God said, "Let Us make man in Our image, according to Our likeness; and let them rule over the fish of the sea and over the birds of the sky and over the cattle and over all the earth, and over every creeping thing that creeps on the earth." God created man in His own image, in the image of God He created him; male and female He created them. (Genesis 1:26-27)

God spoke the heavens and earth into existence. He said, "Let there be..." and it was so. Yet, when it came to man, God didn't speak humanity into existence; He took his time and formed man. God the Father said, let Us make man in Our image, according to Our likeness. God took the time to fashion each cell, DNA, vessel, muscle, organ, and appendages such as eyes, ears, nose, and mouth. Elohim created every hair on man's head, every intricate detail, all the way down to the fingerprints from the dust of the earth. When God looked at Adam's body, He did not say, "and it was good," until He breathed life into his nostrils. When life entered Adams lifeless body, his heart's ventricles began to open and close, allowing blood to circulate throughout the veins and arteries to the whole body, the first heartbeat. The alveoli, air sacs of the lungs were filled with life; oxygen was sent to every part of the body, the first breath. Muscles began to contract, the first movement. Man BECAME a living being. Man was made in the image of God the Father, Son, and Holy Spirit, an image-bearer. God saw all that He had made, and behold, it was very good.

The human body is fascinating. For centuries, scientists have tried to figure out exactly how it works. New discoveries are still being made. I remember sitting in anatomy class, being overwhelmed, trying to learn the intricate details of the muscles, bones, tendons, ligaments, and fascia. This did not even include the immune system, biochemistry, physiology, how the organs functioned alone and in tandem with each other and what happens during the disease processes. Thank the Lord; I made it through medical school. I cannot say I know it all, far from that. I am still being educated and learning something new on a regular basis. This brings me to the human microbiome. In recent years, our understanding of the human microbiome has grown extensively. The body is estimated to contain 100 trillion microbes, which are referred to as the microbiome or microbiota. The human microbiome is composed of bacteria, fungi and viruses. These bacteria, fungi, and viruses help develop our immunity, help us defend ourselves against pathogens. They play a role in nutrition by synthesizing vitamins, producing short-chain fatty acids, and storing fat. The microbiota also has the ability to influence our behavior. The human microbiome is now considered an organ. The microbiota colonizes the skin, mouth and gut. Since the large intestine is the site of the greatest number of microbes and has the greatest diversity, we will take a deeper look into this area. It is estimated to have 10^{11} bacteria/g of colon contents. The gut microbiota is influenced by diet, where you live, age, stress, environmental toxins, antibiotic use, medications, supplements, and disease. As a naturopathic doctor, I consider the health of the intestine with every patient. We believe that most illnesses start in the gut. When the gut is restored, health follows.

Healthy Colon

A healthy colon consists of a diverse group of beneficial bacteria such as: lactobacillus, enterococcus, E. coli, Bifidobacterium, and Bacteroides fragilis. These beneficial bacteria have valuable roles that contribute to health. They help make vitamins, digest fiber, protein, and carbohydrates.

Beneficial bacteria within the gastrointestinal tract are also believed to play a protective role. They protect us by not allowing harmful bacteria, viruses, or fungi to proliferate and lead to disease. As we age, the number of gut bacteria and the diversity of gut bacteria decreases. The bifidobacterial species declines while streptococci, staphylococci, enterococci, and enterobacteria increases.

Unhealthy Colon

An unhealthy colon occurs when there is an imbalance between good and bad bacteria in the intestine; this is called dysbiosis. This imbalance can be caused by diet, age, and antibiotic use. If you are prescribed antibiotics, please take probiotics while on the antibiotic and several weeks after the antibiotic is completed. The antibiotic will kill the good bacteria along with the bad. This practice will help replenish good bacteria and decrease the chances of dysbiosis. I suggest using spore probiotics because the antibiotic will not kill them.

Intestinal Health and COVID-19

You may be wondering how intestinal health relates to COVID-19. Well, the coronavirus has actually been found in stool samples from patients who tested positive for the virus. There have only been a few studies done looking at the microbiome of patients with COVID-19, yet the findings are quite interesting. These studies show that the microorganisms in the gut and lungs of these patients had been altered. These alterations may have a serious impact on the immunity and severity of the virus. An observational study done in China showed that many Chinese patients with the coronavirus had very low levels of two beneficial bacteria: Lactobacillus and Bifidobacterium. Other studies showed a decrease in beneficial gut bacteria, a decrease in bacterial diversity, and an increase in opportunistic pathogens. Opportunistic pathogens are microbes that have the ability to cause disease if given an opportunity. The opportunistic pathogens found were in the fungus family: Candida albicans, Candida auris, and Aspergillus flavus. Another study tested the gut microbiome of 15 patients hospitalized for COVID-19. The results showed that there was a decrease in beneficial bacteria and that patients who had high levels of Clostridium ramosum, and Clostridia hathewayi (opportunistic pathogens) had very severe cases of COVID-19. The results also revealed that when most patients tested negative for COVID-19, they were still deficient in beneficial bacteria. This then leads to the question: could this be a reason why many people who were infected by the virus were still having lingering symptoms after they have recovered?

The Handbook of COVID-19 Prevention and Treatment was published on March 18, 2020, by the First Affiliated Hospital of Zhejiang University School of Medicine. It states in the handbook that, "Some COVID-19 patients have gastrointestinal symptoms (such as abdominal pain and diarrhea) due to direct viral infection of the intestinal mucosa There has been reports that the intestinal microecological *(microbiome)* balance is broken in COVID-19 patients, manifesting a significant reduction of the intestinal probiotics such as lactobacillus and bifidobacterium. Intestinal microecological *(microbiome)* imbalance may lead to bacterial translocation and secondary infection, so it is important to maintain the balance of intestinal microecology by microecological modulator and nutritional support."

Whew, that was a mouthful. Let's break this down. Basically, the doctors in China found that intestinal health plays a very important role in COVID-19 infections. It has been reported that intestinal imbalance has been seen in patients with coronavirus and that when this imbalance occurs, this increases the chances of having secondary infections. The Chinese doctors recommend maintaining intestinal health by taking probiotics. The handbook also says, probiotics and nutritional support should be prescribed to improve gastrointestinal symptoms of patients who are experiencing diarrhea due to COVID-19 to maintain intestinal balance.

Another important point is, as we age, bifidobacterial species decline, which is also what was seen in patients with the Coronavirus. Could this be another reason why older adults are more susceptible to the virus?

Lung Microbiome

Not only do the intestine have a microbiome, the lungs also have a microbiome. In the past, it was thought that the lungs were sterile and did not contain microbiota, but this is far from the truth. Research shows that the lung microbiome helps shape pulmonary immunity by preventing the invasion of pathogens, prevent viruses from attaching to cells and by preventing harmful pathogens from growing when they gain access to the lungs. There is no concrete evidence that the lung microbiome can modify the risk of developing COVID-19 or ARDS, but a couple of studies have been done that show when a person is infected with COVID-19, the lung microbiome changes. In one study, samples of the bronchoalveolar lavage of patients were collected and studied. Eight of the patient samples were positive for COVID-19, 25 had pneumonia, and 20 were used as healthy controls. When the samples were compared, the results showed that there was a significant difference between those with COVID-19 and pneumonia, compared to the samples of healthy patients. Those with infection had elevated levels of pathogenic and commensal bacteria, indicating lung dysbiosis. In another study, lung biopsies were done on patients who had died from COVID-19. The biopsies showed that there were elevated levels of bacteria and fungus found in the lung tissue. Further studies are needed to determine if the lung microbiome plays a part in decreasing the severity of COVID-19 symptoms.

Probiotics

Research shows that probiotics can inhibit the growth of pathogens, modulate the immune system, eliminate toxins from the colon, reduce the incidence, severity and shorten the duration of respiratory tract infections. Because intestinal health is important, and because intestinal imbalances can occur due to diet, age, stress, environmental toxins, medication, etc., it is important that probiotics be a regular part of our routine through food, supplementation, or a combination of both.

Hand Sanitizer / Disinfectants

Among the personal protective equipment suggested to combat COVID-19 is the use of hand sanitizer and disinfectants. People are encouraged to use hand sanitizer when soap and water are not available. Businesses, medical offices, hospitals, churches, restaurants, etc., are required to use disinfectants to sanitize high traffic areas. While this may help decrease the transmittance of the virus, it may have negative long-term effects on the gut microbiome. Disinfectants and sanitizers not only kill viruses; they also kill good bacteria as well. As stated earlier, it is important to have a healthy microbiome, another reason to take probiotics.

Foods

Fermented foods
Unpasteurized Sauerkraut
Pickles (not made with vinegar)
Tempeh
Natto
Miso
Kambucha

Cultured dairy
Yogurt with live or active cultures
Kefir

Recommendations

HMF Forte (Genestra)
HMF Replete (Genestra)
HMF Child (Genestra)
www.DSSOrders.com/DrEdwards
Registration code : VE1366

Spore probiotics (no refrigeration required)
Bacillus coagulans (Thorne)
https://thor.ne/rd6o7

Megasporebiotic (Microbiome labs) Consumer labs found that many supplement companies sold products that did not contain the number of live probiotics stated on the label or were contaminated with "bad" bacteria or mold. The companies I recommend are highly reputable and stand behind their products.

Genesis 2:1-3

Thus the heavens and the earth were completed, and all their hosts.

By the seventh day, God completed His work which He had done, and He rested on the seventh day from all His work which He had done.

Then God blessed the seventh day and sanctified it, because in it He rested from all His work which God had created and made

CHAPTER 15
Day 7

REST

Thus the heavens and the earth were completed, and all their hosts. By the seventh day, God completed His work which He had done, and He rested on the seventh day from all His work which He had done. Then God blessed the seventh day and sanctified it because, in it He rested from all His work which God had created and made (Genesis 2:1-3)

On the seventh day, God rested from all His work and blessed the seventh day and sanctified it. The Hebrew word for rest is ShAvath, it means to repose, desist from exertion, cease, leave off, and come to an end. The primary idea for ShAvath appears to be to sit down or to sit still. Rest in regards to God does not imply that God rested like a weary man but that when God's work was completed and there was no need to continue, He stopped from His creative activity.

The definition of sanctified is to be clean, make clean, hallow, dedicate, consecrate to God, declare as holy, and be regarded as holy. Sanctified signifies an act or a state in which people or things are set aside for use in the worship of God.

In the hustle and bustle of life, do you find that way too often, you are so busy that you don't even have time to eat? Do you take time to just rest? No I am not talking about sleeping but taking personal time for you; that is, time away from the busy schedule of working, going to class, dropping the kids off at practice; time away from the phone, computer, television, iPad, and social media; time, just for you to desist from exertion, to repose, to sit down, or sit still; a time when you just allow things to come to an end? What does that look like in your life? We all got a taste of this when the stay at home order was in place. Did you take advantage of that time to rest or did you just switch from a busy work schedule at the job to a busy work schedule at home? I must admit, the first couple of weeks of working from home, I found myself working more than I would have if I was going into the office. I had to make a conscious effort to stop, reassess and make a change. I had to set boundaries on when I would work and when I would have time to do things that I enjoyed on purpose. Another boundary I had to set was watching the news. At the beginning of the pandemic, I found myself watching the news several times a day to see what the numbers were, how many people were being affected in my hometown, in the US, and all over the world. I would just hear them repeating the same statistics over and over again several times a day. I again had to set a boundary. I made a plan; I would not look at the news several times a day or even daily. And when I did watch it, I would give myself 15-20 minutes to get caught up and then I would shut the TV off.

Please make a conscious effort to set aside time for you; self-care is necessary for your sanity. If God, the creator sets aside time to rest from creating, so can we. We are made in His image, so let's follow His example.

There is a lot going on in 2020. Everyone has been affected in one way or the other by the virus: civil unrest, natural disasters, personal issues, etc. What does REST look like to you? Does this time of rest include curling up with a good book, reading a passage of scripture and meditating on it and allowing it to speak to you, or taking a bath with natural candles burning in the background? Maybe it involves having a massage, listening to your favorite playlist on Spotify or Pandora, walking in the park, sitting at the lake, or kayaking. When it was warm outside, I would go to the lake and work on the manuscript for this book. I saw a couple of ladies kayaking with inflatable kayaks. I struck up a conversation while social distancing and got all the ends and outs about their new-found love. I did some research, as I like to do, and the next week I was on the water with my own inflatable kayak. I absolutely love it. It is relaxing and exhilarating all at the same time, plus I get exercise and vitamin D. Find your thing, and whatever you choose to do; the important thing is that you do it, and you do it regularly.

Part 3

CHAPTER 16

Persistent symptoms after COVID-19

Many people have complaints of lingering symptoms after testing negative for COVID-19.

One study performed in Italy found that weeks after recovery, 87.4% of patients still had at least 1 persistent symptom after testing negative for COVID-19. This study consisted of 143 patients that had recovered from COVID-19, discharged from hospital, out of quarantine, and two negative COVID-19 tests. Patients were assessed approximately 60 days after the onset of the first COVID-19 symptoms. Only 18 of them were completely symptom-free. Forty-four percent reported worsened quality of life, 32% had 1 or 2 symptoms and 55% reported 3 or more symptoms. The top five persistent symptoms reported were fatigue, shortness of breath, joint pains, chest pains, and cough.

Long-term effects of COVID-19 are being seen in children and adults. They are even being seen amongst asymptomatic people. One concern is conditions related to the heart. The risk of heart damage is being experienced by young adults, middle-aged adults, as well as seniors. There may be mild damage to younger people's hearts that will go undetected due to mild symptoms. How this will affect people long-term is unknown. Healthy diets and optimal levels of vitamin C, A, D, zinc, NAC, omega 3's, and probiotics could possibly

prevent persistent long term side
effects from the coronavirus.

Multisystem Inflammatory Syndrome - MIS-C

What is MIS-C?

Many children are being admitted
into the hospital with symptoms
such as fever, low blood pressure,
rash, heart problems, abdominal
pain, gastrointestinal symptoms,
shock, kidney damage, neurological
issues, and several elevated
inflammatory markers. Most do not
have respiratory symptoms;
therefore, in the beginning, these
symptoms were not being related to
COVID-19 until the results showed
that they had antibodies for COVID-
19, indicating recent exposure.

The New England Journal of
Medicine reported that 186 patients
in 26 states have been diagnosed

with Multisystem inflammatory syndrome (MIS-C). Children in other countries are also experiencing these symptoms. It has been reported that approximately 1,000 children worldwide have been diagnosed with MIS-C. In New York, between April 16 and May 4, 2020, 15 children between the ages of 2-15years old were hospitalized for MIS-C, and many were admitted to the intensive care unit. The majority of the children were male and children of color. The children were treated with intravenous immunoglobulins. The majority of them recovered. While many kids will be asymptomatic or have mild side effects from the coronavirus without any persistent side effects, some will not. Be mindful, if your child is having these symptoms and tested negative for the coronavirus test via nose swab, ask if the antibody test can be done to see if that test is positive.

Not only is MIS being seen among children, it is also being seen with adults as well. It has been named MIS-A. Adults are having many of the same symptoms, with little or no respiratory symptoms. Some tested negative for the coronavirus when the test was done via nasal swab. Yet, the antibody test was positive, which indicated coronavirus exposure. A case report involving 16 adults with MIS-A reported that 12 of the patients presented with a fever that lasted longer than 24 hours. Six complained of chest pain or heart palpitations, yet heart irregularities were found in all the patients. Thirteen experienced gastrointestinal symptoms, five had a rash and three had mucositis, inflammation of the mouth mucosa. When x-rays of their lungs were taken, images showed that 10 had pulmonary ground-glass opacities and 6 had pleural effusions, which are common findings among COVID-19 patients. All the patients had elevated inflammatory markers. They were treated with immunoglobulin IV, corticosteroids, tocilizumab, and or interleukin-6 inhibitors. Ten patients were admitted to the ICU, three had to be put on a ventilator, and two died. It is important that if you or a loved one is experiencing these symptoms and has tested negative for the coronavirus, an antibody test should be done to determine past exposure.

CHAPTER 17

Is A Vaccine The Answer?

This section regarding vaccines is not to convince you to take or not to take a vaccine. Its purpose is to arm you with knowledge regarding the body's response to vaccines under certain conditions such as: advanced age, obesity, and nutrient deficiencies.

Operation warp speed has been working since the pandemic started to provide a vaccine against the coronavirus. At this time, there is not a vaccine available. There have been many questions and concerns regarding a vaccine being produced in such a short period of time. Will the vaccine be safe, who will be able to get the vaccine, will there be enough available for everyone who wants to take it? In my research, I came across some very interesting facts regarding current vaccines. I found that there are certain factors that can cause vaccines to be less protective. One study reported that people in advanced age and individuals that are obese have immune systems that don't respond as robustly as younger individuals and those with healthy weight. Therefore, they will have a poorer response to vaccination protection. During the H1N1 pandemic in 2009, studies showed that obese individuals had delayed and weakened immune response to the virus and it took them longer to recover in comparison to healthy weight individuals. It also showed that vaccinated obese individuals have twice the risk of contracting influenza after getting vaccinated compared to healthy weight individuals, indicating poorer protection from the vaccine.

Nutrient deficiencies, such as vitamin A, have been reported to impair vaccination response. Children in Indonesia who were deficient in vitamin A had lower antibody responses when given the tetanus vaccine, compared to those whose vitamin A levels were adequate. Vitamin D also plays a part in how a person responds to vaccines. It has been reported in nine studies involving 2,367 individuals that vitamin D deficiency leads to lower protection from the influenza A and B vaccines. Studies have also shown that people who took probiotics had better responses to vaccines. Having a vaccine readily available will not address the issue fully, when nutrient deficiencies continue to reign in the population. Just as we saw with the stay at home order, it was only part of the solution and when people returned to work, school, etc. the number of cases began to increase. For some reason, healthy nutrition keeps being left out of the equation.

My prayer for you

My prayer is that you and your family will remain in good health during this pandemic. Please implement these simple steps into your daily routine. Getting a good nights sleep, staying well hydrated, eating healthy, and getting sun are foundations to a healthy lifestyle. Adding quality supplementation will help you optimize your immune system during this pandemic. Please share this information with your family and friends.

Beloved, I pray that in all respects you may prosper and be in good health, just as your soul prospers. (3 John 2)

Dr. Vanessa Edwards

Resources

Supplements can also be purchased in the office at:
4421 Salem Ave
Dayton OH 45416

Website:
Vedwardsnd.com

www.DSSOrders.com/DrEdwards
Registration code: VE1366
Coupon code: HCPC1366WELCOME-
10% discount on first order

https://wellevate.me/vanessa-edwards

Liposomal vitamin C (Seeking Health)
Buffered vitamin C (Thorne)
Vitamin A drops (Seeking Health)
Biomins (Thorne)
Meriva (Thorne)
NAC (Seeking Health)
Vitamin D/K2 (Thorne)
Vitamin D3 (Seeking Health

Omega Superb (Thorne)
Super EPA (Thorne)
HMF Forte (Genestra)
HMF Replete (Genestra)
HMF Child (Genestra)
Bacillus coagulans (Thorne)
Megasporebiotic (Microbiome labs)

Blue light blocking glasses
Uvex Skyper Blue Light Blocking Computer
Glasses with SCT-Orange Lens (S1933X)

Want to deepen your walk with God by
fasting?

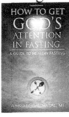

https://amzn.to/2UtTLHB

Acknowlegments

I would like to thank my family, friends,
Pastor Ronald Logan and Sound Words
Christian Education, for your love, support
and encouragement.

About the Author

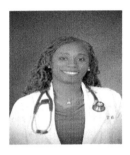

Dr. Vanessa Edwards began her journey of Natural Healing in 1994. She was first trained as a health minister with Hallelujah Acres. At that time, she taught classes and seminars on Nutrition and Health. She then furthered her education by attending medical school at Southwest College of Naturopathic Medicine in Tempe, AZ and received a Master's degree in Chinese Medicine and Acupuncture from Rainstar University and Guan Amen Hospital Beijing, China. Upon graduation, she became the medical director of Arizona Preventive Medicine Clinic in Yuma, AZ. She also opened her own practice in Chandler, AZ, Water of Life Naturopathic Healthcare. In 2008 Dr. Edwards relocated her practice to Dayton OH where she has a thriving practice at the Rapha House Wellness Center. She is also an accomplished conference speaker on health, nutrition and biblical principles.

Dr. Edwards published her first book- How To Get God's Attention In Fasting-A Guide To Healthy Fasting.

Dr. Edwards has volunteered her expertise on many medical missions, offering Naturopathic Healthcare and Acupuncture in: Mexico, Ukraine, Romania, South Africa, Philippines, Dominican Republic, Egypt, Greece, Israel, Rome, Turkey, and Haiti.

Bibliography

A; Nair R; Maseeh. "Vitamin D: The
'Sunshine' Vitamin." *Journal of
Pharmacology & Pharmacotherapeutics*,
U.S. National Library of Medicine, Apr.
2012, pubmed.ncbi.nlm.nih.gov/22629085/.

Agarwal, K S. "The Impact of Atmospheric
Pollution on Vitamin D Status of
Infants and Toddlers in Delhi,
India." *Archives of Disease in
Childhood*, vol. 87, no. 2, 2002, pp.
111–113., doi:10.1136/adc.87.2.111.

Amon, Protima, and Ian Sanderson. "What
Is the Microbiome?" *Archives of
Disease in Childhood - Education &
Practice Edition*, vol. 102, no. 5, 2017,
pp. 257–260.,
doi:10.1136/archdischild-2016-
311643.

"Association of Vitamin D Status and Other
Clinical Characteristics With COVID-
19 Test Results."
doi:10.1107/s0108768107031758/bs5
044sup1.cif.

Balk, R.a. "Benefit of an Enteral Diet
Enriched with Eicosapentaenoic Acid

and Gamma-Linolenic Acid in
Ventilated Patients with Acute Lung
Injury." *Yearbook of Critical Care
Medicine*, vol. 2007, 2007, pp. 225–
226., doi:10.1016/s0734-
3299(08)70366-6.

Bauer, Seth R., et al. "What Is the Role of
Supplementation with Ascorbic Acid,
Zinc, Vitamin D, or N-Acetylcysteine
for Prevention or Treatment of
COVID-19?" *Cleveland Clinic
Journal of Medicine*, Cleveland Clinic
Journal of Medicine, 8 June 2020,
www.ccjm.org/content/early/2020/06/
08/ccjm.87a.ccc046.

Birtolo, Lucia Ilaria, et al. "Coronavirus
Disease 2019 in Rome: Was It
Circulating before
December?" *Journal of
Cardiovascular Medicine*, vol. 21, no.
10, 2020, pp. 835–836.,
doi:10.2459/jcm.0000000000001089.

Bourkhissi, Laila, et al. "Laboratory
Abnormalities in Children with Novel
Coronavirus Disease 2019." *Clinical
Medicine Insights: Pediatrics*, vol. 14,
2020, p. 117955652095517.,
doi:10.1177/1179556520955177.

Carfi, Angelo, et al. "Persistent Symptoms
in Patients After Acute COVID-
19." *Jama*, vol. 324, no. 6, 2020, p.
603., doi:10.1001/jama.2020.12603.

Centers for Disease Control and Prevention,
Centers for Disease Control and
Prevention, 2020, www.cdc.gov/.

Cleveland Clinic Journal of Medicine, 2020,
www.ccjm.org/.

"Data on COVID-19 during
Pregnancy." *Centers for Disease
Control and Prevention*, Centers for
Disease Control and Prevention, Oct.
2020,
www.cdc.gov/coronavirus/2019-
ncov/cases-updates/special-
populations/pregnancy-data-on-covid-
19.html.

David O. Meltzer, MD. "Association of
Vitamin D Status and Other Clinical
Characteristics With COVID-19 Test
Results. *JAMA Network Open*, JAMA
Network, 3 Sept. 2020,
jamanetwork.com/journals/jamanetwo
rkopen/fullarticle/2770157.

Gupta, H., et al. "Potential Use of Turmeric in COVID-19." *Wiley Online Library*, John Wiley & Sons, Ltd, 27 July 2020, onlinelibrary.wiley.com/doi/10.1111/ced.14357.

Horowitz, Richard I., et al. "Efficacy of Glutathione Therapy in Relieving Dyspnea Associated with COVID-19 Pneumonia: A Report of 2 Cases." *Respiratory Medicine Case Reports*, vol. 30, 2020, p. 101063., doi:10.1016/j.rmcr.2020.101063.

"Insufficient Vitamin D Linked to Miscarriage among Women with Prior Pregnancy Loss." *National Institutes of Health*, U.S. Department of Health and Human Services, 4 June 2018, www.nih.gov/news-events/news-releases/insufficient-vitamin-d-linked-miscarriage-among-women-prior-pregnancy-loss.

J;, Pizzorno. "Glutathione!" *Integrative Medicine (Encinitas, Calif.)*, U.S. National Library of Medicine, Feb. 2014, pubmed.ncbi.nlm.nih.gov/26770075/.

Khatiwada, Saroj, and Astha Subedi. "Lung
    Microbiome and Coronavirus Disease
    2019 (COVID-19): Possible Link and
    Implications." *Human Microbiome
    Journal*, vol. 17, 2020, p. 100073.,
    doi:10.1016/j.humic.2020.100073.

Kwok, Yen Lee Angela, et al. "Face
    Touching: A Frequent Habit That Has
    Implications for Hand
    Hygiene." *American Journal of
    Infection Control*, vol. 43, no. 2, 2015,
    pp. 112–114.,
    doi:10.1016/j.ajic.2014.10.015.

Leary, Patrick F., et al. "Effect of Latitude
    on Vitamin D Levels." *The Journal of
    the American Osteopathic Association*,
    vol. 117, no. 7, 2017, p. 433.,
    doi:10.7556/jaoa.2017.089.

Lenton, Kevin J, et al. "Vitamin C
    Augments Lymphocyte Glutathione in
    Subjects with Ascorbate
    Deficiency." *The American Journal of
    Clinical Nutrition*, vol. 77, no. 1,
    2003, pp. 189–195.,
    doi:10.1093/ajcn/77.1.189.

Li, Di Yan. "Melatonin Receptor Genes in
    Vertebrates." *Internet Archive*, 27

May 2013,
archive.org/details/pubmed-
PMC3709728.

Li, Mengmeng, et al. "The SARS-CoV-2
Receptor ACE2 Expression of
Maternal-Fetal Interface and Fetal
Organs by Single Cell Transcriptome
Study." 2020,
doi:10.1101/2020.02.27.967760.

"Listings of WHO's Response to COVID-
19." *World Health Organization*,
World Health Organization, June
2020, www.who.int/news/item/29-06-
2020-covidtimeline.

Loh, Doris. "COVID-19, Pneumonia &
Inflammasomes-the Melatonin
Connection." *Www.evolutamente.it*,
2020, www.evolutamente.it/covid-19-
pneumonia-inflammasomes-the-
melatonin-connection/.

Mazahery, Hajar, and Pamela Von Hurst.
"Factors Affecting 25-
Hydroxyvitamin D Concentration in
Response to Vitamin D
Supplementation." *Nutrients*, vol. 7,
no. 7, 2015, pp. 5111–5142.,
doi:10.3390/nu7075111.

Meltzer, David O., et al. "Association of
Vitamin D Status and Other Clinical
Characteristics With COVID-19 Test
Results." *JAMA Network Open*, vol. 3,
no. 9, 2020,
doi:10.1001/jamanetworkopen.2020.1
9722.

Morris, Sapna Bamrah, et al. "Case Series of
Multisystem Inflammatory Syndrome
in Adults Associated with SARS-
CoV-2 Infection — United Kingdom
and United States, March–August
2020." *MMWR. Morbidity and
Mortality Weekly Report*, vol. 69, no.
40, 2020, pp. 1450–1456.,
doi:10.15585/mmwr.mm6940e1.

Morris, Sapna. "Case Series of Multisystem
Inflammatory Syndrome in Adults
Associated with SARS-CoV-2
Infection - United Kingdom and
United States, March-August
2020." *Centers for Disease Control
and Prevention*, Centers for Disease
Control and Prevention, 8 Oct. 2020,
www.cdc.gov/mmwr/volumes/69/wr/
mm6940e1.htm.

Polonikov, Alexey. "Endogenous
Deficiency of Glutathione as the Most

Likely Cause of Serious
Manifestations and Death in COVID-
19 Patients." *ACS Infectious Diseases*,
vol. 6, no. 7, 2020, pp. 1558–1562.,
doi:10.1021/acsinfecdis.0c00288.

Pontes-Arruda, Alessandro, et al. "Effects of
Enteral Feeding with Eicosapentaenoic
Acid, γ-Linolenic Acid, and
Antioxidants in Mechanically
Ventilated Patients with Severe Sepsis
and Septic Shock*." *Critical Care
Medicine*, vol. 34, no. 9, 2006, pp.
2325–2333.,
doi:10.1097/01.ccm.0000234033.6565
7.b6.

Preiser, Jean-Charles. "Faculty Opinions
Recommendation of Effects of Enteral
Feeding with Eicosapentaenoic Acid,
Gamma-Linolenic Acid, and
Antioxidants in Mechanically
Ventilated Patients with Severe Sepsis
and Septic Shock." *Faculty Opinions –
Post-Publication Peer Review of the
Biomedical Literature*, 2006,
doi:10.3410/f.1046339.496285.

Rogero, Marcelo M., et al. "Potential
Benefits and Risks of Omega-3 Fatty
Acids Supplementation to Patients

with COVID-19." *Free Radical
Biology and Medicine*, Pergamon, 10
July 2020,
www.sciencedirect.com/science/article
/pii/S0891584920311412.

Ryan, Goodman, and Schulkin Danielle.
"Timeline of the Coronavirus
Pandemic and U.S. Response." *Just
Security*, 15 Oct. 2020,
www.justsecurity.org/69650/timeline-
of-the-coronavirus-pandemic-and-u-s-
response/.

Silverman, Justin D., et al. "Using Influenza
Surveillance Networks to Estimate
State-Specific Prevalence of SARS-
CoV-2 in the United States." *Science
Translational Medicine*, American
Association for the Advancement of
Science, 29 July 2020,
stm.sciencemag.org/content/12/554/ea
bc1126.full.

Singer, Pierre, et al. "Benefit of an Enteral
Diet Enriched with Eicosapentaenoic
Acid and Gamma-Linolenic Acid in
Ventilated Patients with Acute Lung
Injury*." *Critical Care Medicine*, vol.
34, no. 4, 2006, pp. 1033–1038.,

doi:10.1097/01.ccm.0000206111.2362
9.0a.

Valenti, Luca, et al. "SARS-CoV-2
Seroprevalence Trends in Healthy
Blood Donors during the COVID-19
Milan Outbreak." 2020,
doi:10.1101/2020.05.11.20098442.

Wu, Zunyou, and Jennifer M. Mcgoogan.
"Characteristics of and Important
Lessons From the Coronavirus
Disease 2019 (COVID-19) Outbreak
in China." *Jama*, vol. 323, no. 13,
2020, p. 1239.,
doi:10.1001/jama.2020.2648.

Ye, Qing, et al. "The Pathogenesis and
Treatment of the `Cytokine Storm' in
COVID-19." *Journal of Infection*, vol.
80, no. 6, 2020, pp. 607–613.,
doi:10.1016/j.jinf.2020.03.037

Made in the USA
Middletown, DE
10 August 2021